PELICAN BOOKS

COGNITIVE THERAPY AND THE EMOTIONAL DISORDERS

Aaron T. Beck is University Professor of Psychiatry at the University of Pennsylvania School of Medicine and Director of its Center for Cognitive Therapy, a world-renowned training centre for the approaches he has developed. A graduate of Brown University, he received his M.D. at the Yale School of Medicine.

Dr Beck is the author of a number of books on depression, anxiety, suicide and cognitive therapy, including *Love is Never Enough*, which is also published in Penguin. He has written over 200 scientific and scholarly articles and monographs and his work has had a major impact on the understanding and treatment of psychological disorders and interpersonal problems. He has received numerous honours for his contributions to psychotherapy, including the Foundation Fund Prize for Research in Psychiatry of the American Psychiatric Association and the Paul Hoch Award of the American Psychopathological Association. In 1982 he received an honorary Doctor of Medical Science degree from Boston University and in 1987 was elected a Fellow of the Royal College of Psychiatrists.

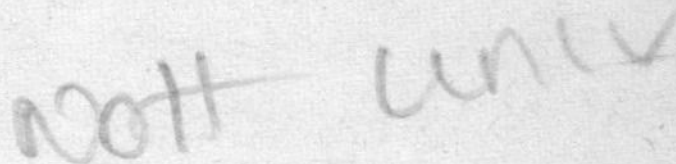

COGNITIVE THERAPY AND THE EMOTIONAL DISORDERS

Aaron T. Beck, M.D.

PENGUIN BOOKS

PENGUIN BOOKS

Published by the Penguin Group
27 Wrights Lane, London W8 5TZ, England
Viking Penguin Inc., 40 West 23rd Street, New York, New York 10010, USA
Penguin Books Australia Ltd, Ringwood, Victoria, Australia
Penguin Books Canada Ltd, 2801 John Street, Markham, Ontario, Canada L3R 1B4
Penguin Books (NZ) Ltd, 182–190 Wairau Road, Auckland 10, New Zealand

Penguin Books Ltd, Registered Offices: Harmondsworth, Middlesex, England

First published in the United States by International Universities Press, Inc. 1976
Published in Penguin Books 1989
1 3 5 7 9 10 8 6 4 2

Published by arrangement with NAL Penguin Inc., New York, New York

Printed and bound in Great Britain by
Cox & Wyman Ltd, Reading

To Phyllis
and
Alice, Daniel, Judy, and Roy

Contents

Introduction

In recent years, emotional disorders have attracted an enormous amount of attention and publicity. This intense interest is readily evident in the best-seller list of books sold to the public and in the contents of popular magazines. College courses in abnormal psychology have achieved a spectacular growth in popularity, and the number of psychiatrists, clinical psychologists, and other professionals in the mental health field has escalated. Bountiful outlays of public funds, as well as private contributions, have been poured into an enormous expansion of community mental health centers and other psychiatric facilities.

Paradoxically, the popularization of emotional disorders and the prodigious efforts to mass-produce professional services have occurred in the context of increasingly sharp disagreements among authorities regarding the nature and appropriate treatment of these disorders. With intriguing regularity, new theories and therapies have captured the imagination of both the layman and the professional and have then gradually drifted into oblivion. Moreover, the most durable schools devoted to the study and treatment of emotional disturbances—traditional neuropsychiatry, psychoanalysis, and behavior therapy—still retain their original differences in theoretical framework and experimental and clinical approaches.

Despite the striking differences among these dominant schools, they share one basic assumption: The emotionally disturbed person is victimized by concealed forces over which he has no control. Emerging from the nineteenth-century doctrine of physicalism, traditional neuropsychiatry searches for biological causes such as chemical or neurological abnormalities, and applies drugs and other physical measures to relieve the emotional disorder. Psychoanalysis, whose philosophical underpinnings also were formed in the nineteenth century, attributes an individual's neurosis to unconscious psychological factors: The unconscious elements are sealed off by psychological barriers that can only be penetrated by psychoanalytic interpretations. Behavior therapy, whose philosophical roots can be traced to the eighteenth century, regards the emotional disturbance in terms of involuntary reflexes based on accidental conditionings that occurred previously in the patient's life. Since, according to behavioral theory, the patient cannot modify these conditioned reflexes simply by knowing about them and trying to will them away, he requires the application of "counterconditioning" by a competent behavior therapist.

Because these three leading schools maintain that the source of the patient's disturbance lies beyond his awareness, they gloss over his conscious conceptions, his specific thoughts and fantasies.

Suppose, however, that these schools are on the wrong track. Let us conjecture, for the moment, that a person's consciousness contains elements that are responsible for the emotional upsets and blurred thinking explanations are regarded as spurious rationalizations, his coping mechanisms as defenses. Consequently, his conscious ideas, his reasoning and judgements, his practical solutions to problems are not taken at face value: they are treated as stepping-stones to deeper, concealed components of the mind.

The behavior therapists, similarly, have tended to downgrade the importance of thinking, but for completely different reasons. In their zeal to emulate the precision and theoretical elegance of the physical sciences, the original behaviorists rejected data and concepts derived from man's reflections on his conscious experiences. Only behavior that could be directly observed by an independent outsider was used in forming explanations. Hence, thoughts, feelings, and ideas, which, by definition, are accessible only to the person experiencing them, were not considered valid data. The patient's private world was not regarded as a useful area of inquiry (Watson, 1914; Skinner, 1971).

Traditional neuropsychiatry, like psychoanalysis and behavior therapy, also minimizes the importance of conscious ideation. The neuropsychiatrist, sometimes referred to as an "organicist," inquires about the patient's thoughts and feelings primarily as a basis for making a diagnosis. Abnormal ideation and feeling states are regarded simply as manifestations of an underlying physical process or as possible clues to a disturbance in neurochemistry; they are not explored to provide explanations for abnormal psychological states.

Proponents of the three major schools use therap in keeping with their philosophical and theor origins. The Freudian, with his belief in depth psyc and symbolic meanings, attempts to cure the neu uncovering the hidden (that is, repressed) ideas and wishes and by translating the conscious thoughts and fantasies into their presumed symbolic meanings. The behavior therapist, with his faith in the determinative role of environmental (that is, observable) forces, attempts to enucleate the neurosis through external stimuli: administering rewards and punishments, exposing the patient by degrees to situations or objects that frighten him. The neuropsychiatrist, with his confidence in the role of biological causes, uses "somatic" treatments such as the administration of drugs or electroconvulsive therapy.

By glossing over the patient's attempts to define his problem in his own terms, and the efficacy of using his own rationality to solve his problems, the contemporary schools perpetuate a myth. The troubled person is led to believe that he can't help himself and must seek out a professional healer when confronted with distress related to everyday problems of living. His confidence in the "obvious" techniques he has customarily used in solving his problems is eroded because he accepts the view that emotional disturbances arise from forces beyond his grasp. He can't hope to understand himself through his own efforts because his own notions are dismissed as shallow and insubstantial: By debasing the value of common sense, this subtle indoctrination inhibits him from using his own judgment in analyzing and solving his problems. This pervasive attitude also deters the psychotherapist from helping the patient to draw on his own problem-solving apparatus.

Other writers have been concerned about the tendency to ignore the importance of common-sense psychology. Allport (1968) for example, once remarked,

"How in the helping professions—and here I include psychiatry, the ministry, social work, applied psychology, and education—can we recover some of the common sense that we seem to have lost along the way?" (p. 125). The professional's inattentiveness to the patient's conscious ideas and coping techniques has been appropriately captioned "blind to the obvious" by Icheiser (1970, p. 7).

CONSCIOUSNESS AND COMMON SENSE

When we consider the complexities and pressures of everyday life, we can only marvel that our fellow man is able to function as well as he does. He not only adapts to helter-skelter changes in his environment and difficult confrontations with other people, but he also manages to negotiate numerous compromises between his own wishes, hopes, and expectations, on the one hand, and external demands and constraints, on the other. Disappointments, frustrations, criticisms are absorbed without lasting damage.

Modern man is often forced to make extremely rapid life-and-death decisions (as when driving a car). He makes even more difficult judgments in distinguishing circumstances that actually are dangerous from those that simply *seem* dangerous (for example, distinguishing between a genuine threat and a bluff).

If it were not for man's ability to filter and attach appropriate labels to the blizzard of external stimuli so efficiently, his world would be chaotic and he would be bounced from one crisis to another. Moreover, if he were not able to monitor his highly developed imagination, he would be floating in and out of a twilight zone unable to distinguish between the reality of a situation and the images and personal meanings that it triggers.

In his interpersonal relations, he is generally able to select the subtle cues that allow him to separate his adversaries from his friends. He makes the delicate adjustments in his own behavior that help him to maintain diplomatic relationships with people whom he dislikes or who dislike him. He is generally able to penetrate the social masks of other people, to differentiate sincere from insincere messages, to distinguish friendly mocking from veiled antagonism. He tunes into the significant communications in a vast babble of noises so that he can organize and modulate his own responses. These psychological operations seem to work automatically without evidence of much cognition, deliberation, or reflection.

These observations provide powerful evidence that, in the course of our development, we have acquired highly refined, sophisticated techniques for dealing with the intricacies of our animate and inanimate environment. Moreover, we have within the range of our awareness a vast reservoir of information, concepts, and formulas that enable us to deal with our familiar psychological problems. Of course, we make mistakes in appraising a situation and our own capabilities; we encounter many problems for which we have no ready-made solutions and are often required to make decisions without having been provided with adequate information. Nonetheless, we are able to use our psychological equipment to make split-second corrections, to judge, interpret, and predict. We can approach new problems in a systematic way, separate the various components, and consider alternative solutions.

In his approach to external problems, man is a practical scientist: He makes observations, sets up hypotheses, checks their validity, and eventually forms generalizations that will later serve as a guide for making rapid judgments of situations. Although much of his early learning is based on trial-and-error and inductive reasoning, he is able to accumulate an inventory of formulas, equations, and axioms that enable him to make rapid deductions when confronted with the same kinds of problems that he has already worked out. Throughout his development, man repeatedly uses the prototype of the experimental method—without recognizing it.

In the area of strictly psychological problems, a person acquires a host of techniques and generalizations that enable him to judge whether he is reacting realistically to situations, to resolve conflicts regarding alternative courses of actions, to deal with rejection, disappointment, and danger. In the course of development, his awareness of his own psychological experiences crystallizes into defined self-observations, which eventually expand into generalizations. As these improvised techniques stand the test of time, they provide the framework for genuine self-understanding and understanding of others. As we shall see, much of cognitive therapy places the patient in the role of the scientist and uses his already-available tools to approach problems that seemed insoluble to him.

Fortunately, each person does not have to start *de novo* in acquiring such understandings. Through the process of socialization he receives a rich infusion of folk wisdom: axioms of human behavior and homespun logic. By virtue of his personal experience, emulation of others, and formal education, he learns how to use the tools of common sense: forming and testing hunches, making discriminations, and reasoning. The wise person is able to extract the sound principles from the thick brew of his cultural heritage and to ignore the residue of fallacious notions, myths, and superstitions.

The significance of common sense extends far beyond social learning. The importance of common sense in formal science, for example, has long been recognized by scientists and philosophers. The introductory quotation of Whitehead is echoed by J. Robert Oppenheimer (1956): "All sciences . . . arise as refinements, corrections, and adaptations of common sense" (p. 128).

Observations of *external* events—and common-sense laws based on these observations—were the starting point for physics and chemistry. The common-sense observation that unsupported bodies will fall was the necessary precursor to the laws of gravity; that water heated over a flame for a sufficient length of time will boil, to laws of heat and gases. Similarly, observations of consciousness—that is, of *internal* psychological events—provide the raw materials for the systematic study of human behavior.

The implications of common sense for the development of a scientific psychology have been extensively discussed by Heider (1958). As he indicates, the complexity of feelings and actions that can be understood at a glance is surprisingly great. "Intuitive" knowledge is remarkably penetrating and can go a long way toward the understanding of human behavior. Heider points out, "The ordinary person has a great and profound understanding of himself and of other people which, though unformulated or only vaguely conceived, enables him to interact with others in more or less adaptive ways" (p. 2).

Common-sense psychology includes the psychological operations, reflections, observations, and introspections by which someone attempts to determine why he is upset, what is bothering him, and what he can do to relieve his distress. Through introspection, he can determine the main topic of his ideation and relate this to his unpleasant feelings (tension, sadness, irritation). The person also uses common-sense psychology when he attempts to identify the events or circumstances that have triggered his particular preoccupation, and consequently his distress. Moreover, he can then take measures to relieve his pain.

This kind of ordinary self-help is frequently applied to understanding and helping others; for example, encouraging them to focus on what is bothering them and then suggesting more sensible attitudes or more realistic solutions to problems. It is obvious that conveying commonplace understandings and giving practical advice does not always work, but it seems to help many, perhaps most, people to maintain their equilibrium most of the time. Furthermore, these common-sense insights and interpersonal strategies point the way to the development of a sophisticated, systematic psychotherapy.

WHEN COMMON SENSE FAILS

Despite the obvious value of common sense as a framework for understanding and changing attitudes and behavior, we are all familiar with its shortcomings: Common sense has failed to provide plausible and useful explanations for the puzzling emotional disorders.

Take, for example, the riddle of depression: A depressed woman who always had a great zest for life, had felt a great deal of pride in herself and in her achievements, and had cared for her children with obvious love and tenderness, became morose and lost interest in everything that had previously excited her. She withdrew into a shell, neglected her children, and became preoccupied with self-criticisms and wishes to die. At one point, she formulated a plan to kill herself and her children, but was stopped before she could carry out the plan.

How can conventional folk wisdom explain this woman's remarkable change from her normal state? In common with other depressed patients, she appears to violate the most basic principles of human nature. Her suicidal wishes and her desire to kill her children defy the most hallowed "survival instinct" and "maternal instinct." Her withdrawal and self-debasements are clear-cut contradictions of another accepted canon of human behavior—the pleasure principle. Common sense is foiled in attempting to understand and to fit together the components of her depression. Sometimes the deep suffering and withdrawal of the patient is explained away by conventional notions such as, "He is just trying to get attention." The notion that a person tortures himself to the point of suicide for the dubious satisfaction of gaining attention greatly strains our credulity and actually runs counter to common sense.

In order to understand why the depressed mother would want to end her own life and that of her children, we need to get inside her conceptual system and see the world through her eyes. We cannot be bound by preconceptions that are applicable to people who are not depressed. Once we are familiar with the perspectives of the depressed patient, her behavior begins to make sense.

Through a process of empathy and identification with the patient, we can understand the meanings she attaches to her experiences. We can then offer explanations that are plausible—given her frame of reference.

Through interviewing this depressed mother, I discovered that her thinking was controlled by erroneous ideas about herself and her world. Despite contrary evidence, she believed she had been a failure as a mother. She viewed herself as too incompetent to provide even the minimum care and affection for her children. She believed that she could not change—but could only deteriorate. Since she could attribute her presumed failure and inadequacy only to herself, she tormented herself continuously with self-rebukes.

As this depressed woman visualized the future, she expected her children would feel as miserable as she. Casting about for solutions, she decided that since she could not change, the only answer was suicide. Yet, she was appalled at the notion that her children would be left without a mother, without the love and care she believed that only a mother could give. Consequently, she decided that in order to spare them the kind of misery she was experiencing, she must end their lives also. It is noteworthy that these self-deceptions dominated the patient's consciousness but were not elicited until she was carefully questioned about her thoughts and plans.

This kind of depressive thinking may strike us as highly irrational, but it makes sense within the patient's conceptual framework. If we grant her the basic (though erroneous) premise, namely that she and her children are irrevocably doomed as a result of her presumed deficiencies, it follows logically that the sooner the situation is terminated the better for everyone. Her basic premise of being inadequate and incapable of doing anything accounts for her complete withdrawal and loss of motivation. Her feelings of overwhelming sadness stem inevitably from her continous self-criticisms and her belief that her present and future are hopeless. Having pinpointed the exact content of the patient's erroneous beliefs, I was able to draw on a variety of methods to correct her misconceptions and to induce her to examine the unrealistic premises of her belief system.

This example demonstrates why common sense has failed to clarify emotional disorders such as depression. Crucial information (in this case, the patient's distorted view of herself, her world, and her future) is lacking. However, *once the missing data are supplied*, we can apply common-sense tools to solve the puzzle. As we fit the relevant material into place, a comprehensible, meaningful pattern emerges. In order to draw reliable generalizations from this finding, we check for the presence of this kind of pattern in other patients with the same emotional disorder. Then it is necessary to conduct a logical sequence of experimental procedures to consolidate the new framework for understanding the particular disorder. After the experimental findings have been checked, refined, and validated, we can test our formulation against Whitehead's ultimate requirement: Does it satisfy common sense?

Consider the case of the compulsive hand-washer. He spends inordinate amounts of time scrubbing his hands and other exposed parts of his body. When pressed for an explanation, he may state that he is concerned because he may have come into contact with germs that could produce a serious disease if he is not thoroughly cleansed. He may even acknowledge that this fear is far-fetched, yet he continues with his handwashing even though it seriously interferes with his career, social relations, and recreation—even his sleeping and eating. The classical psychoanalytic explanation of this kind of behavior is that the patient has an anal fixation or that he is trying to wash away the guilt stemming from some forbidden, but unconscious, wish.

When the patient's thinking is thoroughly explored, however, the following facts are revealed: We learn that whenever he touches an object that might contain bacteria, he has the thought that he may contract a bad disease. At the same time, he has a *visual image* of himself in a hospital bed dying from this disease. The thought and visual fantasy produce anxiety. In order to counteract and dampen his fear, he rushes to the nearest washroom to start scrubbing himself.

In treating such cases, I have set up a procedure of inducing the patient to touch a dirty object in my presence, but—by prior agreement—I eliminate the opportunity for his washing his hands. Deprived of the mechanism for ridding himself of the supposed germ-laden dirt, he begins to visualize himself in the hospital bed, dying of the dread disease. This visual fantasy comes on spontaneously and is so vivid that the patient believes that he already has the disease: He starts to cough, feels feverish and weak, and experiences peculiar sensations throughout his body. By interrupting his visual fantasy, I can demonstrate to him that he is not sick: He still has his strength, does not have a fever, and can breathe without coughing. The sequence of interrupting his visual image and prodding him to make a realistic appraisal of his state of health relieves his fear of having contracted a fatal disease and reduces his compulsion to wash his hands.

Having ferreted out the crucial information, namely that this patient experiences a fantasy and a physical experience of having a serious disease if prevented from cleansing himself, we find that his hand-washing compulsion is comprehensible. Furthermore, this information relieves us of the temptation to grasp for some esoteric interpretation that will not help the patient with his serious psychological problem. The compulsive hand-washer illustrates what a crucial role imaginal processes, including both visual fantasies and the accompanying physical sensations based on self-suggestion, play in certain disorders.

BEYOND COMMON SENSE: COGNITIVE THERAPY

The formulation of psychological problems in terms of incorrect premises and a proneness to distorted imaginal experiences represents a sharp deviation from generally accepted formulations of the psychological disorders. Freud assumed that peculiar behavior has its roots in the Unconscious, and that any irrationalities observed on the conscious level are only manifestations of the underlying unconscious drives. The presence of self-deception and distortions, however, does not require the postulation of the unconscious, as conceived by Freud. Irrationality can be understood in terms of inadequacies in organizing and interpreting reality.

Psychological problems are not necessarily the product of mysterious, impenetrable forces but may result from commonplace processes such as faulty learning, making incorrect inferences on the basis of inadequate or incorrect information, and not distinguishing adequately between imagination and reality. Moreover, thinking can be unrealistic because it is derived from erroneous premises; behavior can be self-defeating because it is based on unreasonable attitudes.

Thus, psychological problems can be mastered by sharpening discriminations, correcting misconceptions, and learning more adaptive attitudes. Since introspection, insight, reality testing, and learning are basically cognitive processes, this approach to the neuroses has been labeled cognitive therapy (Beck, 1967, p. 318).

The cognitive therapist induces the patient to apply the same problem-solving techniques he has used throughout his life to correct his fallacious thinking. His problems are derived from certain distortions of reality based on erroneous premises and misconceptions. These distortions originated in defective learning during his development. The formula for treatment may be stated in simple terms: The therapist helps the patient to identify his warped thinking and to learn more realistic ways to formulate his experiences.

The cognitive approach brings the understanding and treatment of the neurotic disorders closer to everyday experience. Emotional disturbances can be related to the kinds of misunderstandings a person has experienced numerous times during his life. Since the psychiatric patient has generally had numerous previous successes in correcting his misinterpretations, the cognitive approach makes sense to him because it is in line with his previous learning experiences. By placing emotional disorders within the realm of everyday experience and suggesting familiar problem-solving techniques, the therapist can start to help the patient at the time of their first contact.

Recent developments within the major schools of psychology and psychotherapy attest to the importance of cognitive psychology in understanding and treating the neuroses. The growing confluence of tributaries from behavioral psychology and psychoanalysis has been charted by Robert Holt (1964). The behaviorists and psychoanalysts have become aware that there are legitimate and important problems left unsolved by their neglect of the cognitive realm. The psychoanalysts, who strove for depth, and the behaviorists, who prized objectivity above all else, have begun to realize that they do not have to betray their basic values to study these problems. Ego psychology began to emerge within psychoanalysis as a result of the stimulus of writers such as Hartmann (1964), Kris (1952), and Rapaport (1951). Attention was directed to the nature of reality and man's adaptation to it. Learning has always been a central concern of the behaviorists; gradually, they have shown an interest in thinking and thought processes, learning concepts as well as motor performances, learning words as well as nonsense syllables.

Despite their continued allegiance to their respective schools, many practitioners are increasingly using cognitive techniques in their treatment of patients. Much of behavior therapy, for instance, while ostensibly derived from laboratory experiments and from learning theory, is to a large degree an assortment of time-honored techniques used by people to deal with their psychological problems. Rehearsing frightening situations in fantasy in order to reduce fear of a relatively innocuous situation (the core of the behavioral technique of "systematic desensitization") and practicing self-assertion ("assertive training") have been independently improvised by numerous people for ages. Similarly, many neuropsychiatrists, without abandoning their notion of physical causation, prescribe a variety of practical remedies for neurosis: re-education and explanation, encouragement, and environmental change.

The growth of this common ground may very well be enhanced by the spirited endeavors of humanistic psychologists and psychiatrists who have been dubbed "the third force" (Goble, 1970). This change of focus to a person's conscious thoughts, wishes, and ideals has been hailed by Allport (1968) as "a significant revolution." Referring to this approach as "attitudinal" therapy, he perceives points of congruence in the theories of such diverse writers as Adler, Erikson, Horney, Maslow, and Rogers. The work of Albert Ellis should be added to this list.

What is this middle ground that has been staked out by "third-force" humanists and that is gradually being watered by spillovers from psychoanalysis and behaviorism? Their approach consists of greater interest in, and willingness to accept at face value, conscious thoughts, goals, and attitudes. These theorists focus on the person's ideas—his introspections, his observations of himself, his plans for solving problems.

The crucial importance of cognitive psychology as a way of understanding human problems has been underscored by Arieti (1968), a psychoanalyst who has called cognition the "Cinderella" of the field of psychiatry. He emphasizes that, "A great deal of human life has to do with conceptual constructs. It is impossible to understand the human being without such important cognitive constructs as the self-image, self-esteem, self-identity, identification, hope, projection of the self into the future" (p. 1637).

Because cognitive phenomena are easily identified through introspection, they may be readily investigated. The accessibility of the patient's cognitions to systematic investigation has attracted many behaviorally trained writers (for example, Mahoney, 1974; Meichenbaum, 1974) to explore the role of cognitive processes in psychopathology and psychotherapy. Recent systematic studies have provided large areas of support for the principles of cognitive therapy. Finally, the increasing interest in this approach has led to a number of therapeutic trials that have indicated the efficacy of cognitive therapy.

CHAPTER 2

Tapping the Internal Communications

A personality is a full Congress of orators and pressure-groups, of children, demagogues, communists, isolationists, war-mongers, mugwumps, grafters, log-rollers, lobbyists, Caesars and Christs, Machiavels and Judases, Tories and Promethean revolutionists. —Henry Murray

THE HIDDEN MESSAGE

We are all aware of the various ways that the signs and signals from our environment dictate what we do and how we feel. We stop at red lights, detour blasting areas, protest over mistreatment, exult over praise, and grouse over reproaches. We are less familiar with the internal organization of signals that correspond to external signals. Incoming messages are processed, decoded, and interpreted by our self-regulating system that issues instructions and prohibitions, self-praise and self-reproaches.

The complex system of environmental stimuli controls us only to the extent that it meshes with its internal psychological counterpart. Our inner workings can shut out or twist around the signals from the outside so that we may be completely out of phase with what is going on around us. A profound or chronic discrepancy between the internal and the external systems may culminate in psychological disorders.

Many of the characteristics of the emotional disorders are puzzling and seem to defy common-sense laws because of the poverty of relevant information. When the missing data are supplied, the investigator or therapist can readily apply his tools to make sense out of the most perplexing behaviors. Unraveling the meanings woven into an anomolous reaction is an intriguing enterprise that provides a wealth of insight into human behavior. Consider these representative examples from clinical practice:

A woman walking out-of-doors suddenly realized that she was about three blocks from home and immediately felt faint.

A professional athlete consistently felt his chest constrict and his heart pound whenever he was driving his automobile through a tunnel. He started to gasp for breath and thought he was dying.

A successful novelist cried bitterly when he was complimented for his work.

Puzzling reactions such as these have stimulated various schools of psychotherapy to reach into their conceptual baggage for explanations. Psychoanalysis, for example, has explained a woman's feeling faint when away from home in terms of unconscious meaning: Being out-of-doors stirs up a repressed desire such as a wish for seduction or rape (Fenichel, 1945). The wish arouses anxiety because of its taboo nature.

Behaviorists, on the other hand, using a conditioning model of emotions to account for the anxiety, provide a different kind of explanation. They assume that at some time in the woman's life she was confronted with a realistically dangerous situation, while simultaneously being exposed to an innocuous situation (such as traveling away from home). Because of the closeness of the innocuous stimulus to the real danger, the woman became conditioned to react to the innocuous stimulus with as much anxiety as she would experience in the face of a real danger (Wolpe, 1969).

The psychoanalytic and behaviorist explanations of the woman's anxiety are dictated by theory and do not take advantage of all the relevant data. Another explanation forces itself upon us when we tap the internal communication system.

Each of the patients described above was aware of having had a sequence of thoughts that intervened between the event and the unpleasant emotional reaction. When a person is able to fill in the gap between an activating event and the emotional consequences, the puzzling reaction becomes understandable. With training, people are able to catch the rapid thoughts or images that occur between an event and the emotional response.

The woman observed the following chain of ideas immediately before she became anxious. As soon as she became aware that she was several blocks from her house, she would think, "I am really far away from home. If something happened to me now, I couldn't get back in time to get help. If I fell down on the street here, people would just walk by—they wouldn't know me. Nobody would help me." The chain of events leading to anxiety included a sequence of thoughts of danger.

The athlete with the tunnel phobia also was able to identify a specific series of ideas revolving about the concept of danger. As he entered the tunnel, he would think, "This tunnel could collapse and I would suffocate." He then had a visual image of these dire happenings and immediately began to experience tension in his chest—which he interpreted as a sign that he was suffocating. The thoughts of suffocation generated further anxiety which was manifested by an increased pulse rate and shortness of breath.

The novelist, who was in the throes of a depression, reacted to a compliment about his writing with this procession of thoughts: "People won't be honest with me. They *know* that I'm mediocre. They just won't accept me as I really am. They keep giving me phony compliments." When he revealed these thoughts, his adverse reaction to praise became intelligible: Since he regarded his work as inferior, he interpreted positive statements as being insincere. His erroneous conclusion that he could not have a genuine relationship with other people made him feel more isolated and more depressed.

The principle that there is a conscious thought between an external event and a particular emotional response is not generally accepted by the major schools of psychotherapy. Their exclusion of conscious ideation from their theoretical formulations is an inevitable consequence of not investigating this crucial source of information. It is not difficult, however, to train subjects or patients to focus on their introspections in various situations. The person can then observe that a thought links the external stimulus with the emotional response.

We know that a person may suddenly experience an emotion when there is no external event to account for it. In such instances, it is usually possible to ascertain that there is an integral "cognitive event" (that is, a thought, a reminiscence, image, in his free-flowing stream of consciousness) which produced the emotional response. In emotional disturbances such as depression or anxiety neurosis this prevailing cognitive flow may account for the persistent unpleasant emotions.

Many behavioral scientists object to the concept that ideation plays a crucial role in shaping emotional responses. Some argue that the emotional response is triggered directly by the external stimuli and that the person inserts his cognitive appraisal of the event only retrospectively. A person who is trained to track his thoughts, however, can observe repeatedly that his interpretation of a situation *precedes* his emotional response to it. For example, he sees a car heading toward him; then, he thinks, "It is going to hit me," and feels anxious. Furthermore, when a person changes his appraisal of a situation, his emotional reaction changes. A young woman believed that a friend passed by her without saying hello. She thought, "He's snubbing me," and felt sad. After a second glance, she realized that it wasn't her friend at all and her hurt feelings disappeared.

In fact, it is difficult to conceive of how a person can react emotionally to an event before he has appraised its nature. The significant details in his environment, unlike simple laboratory stimuli such as a ringing bell or dermal shocks used in many behavioral experiments, are generally complex. Judgment is required to decide whether a situation is safe or harmless, whether another person is friendly or unfriendly: Often a subtle clue determines whether he is joking or being hostile. If not for cognitive processes such as discrimination and integration of stimuli, we would react willy-nilly to events. Whether we laughed, cried, or raged would have no sensible relation to the reality of what was happening. Such capricious responses might be predicted from behavior theory, which asserts that emotional responses are based on accidental past conditionings and set off by the occurrence of events that had been associated by chance with emotionally arousing situation in the past.

The importance of eliciting a person's cognitions becomes apparent when we attempt to understand incongruous emotional reactions. We find that apparently unrealistic or exaggerated anger, anxiety, or sadness is based on the individual's peculiar appraisal of the event. These peculiar appraisals become dominant in emotional disorders.

THE DISCOVERY OF AUTOMATIC THOUGHTS

My formulation of the role of cognition in emotional disorders and in psychotherapy may be explained further by an autobiographical note. I had been practicing psychoanalysis and psychoanalytic psychotherapy for many years before I was struck by the fact that a patient's cognitions had an enormous impact on his feelings and behavior. All my patients had been instructed in the basic rule of free association ("The patient is requested to say everything that enters his mind, without selection" [Fenichel, 1945, p. 23]) and most learned quite well to overcome the tendency to censor their ideas. They expressed rather freely feelings, wishes, and experiences they had concealed from other people because of fear of disapproval. Although I recognized that my patients could not possibly report all their thoughts, I believed that their verbalizations represented a fairly good cross-section of their conscious ideation.

In time, however, I began to suspect that the patients were not reporting certain kinds of ideation. This omission was not due to any resistance or defensiveness on the part of the patient, but rather it had to do with the fact that the patient had not been trained to focus on certain kinds of thought. In retrospect, it is apparent to me that the types of ideation that had gone unnoticed are in fact crucial to understanding the nature of psychological problems. Although other psychoanalysts may have exposed this rich vein of material, they had not reported it as such in the literature.

The following experience triggered my interest and consequent investigation of this unverbalized material.

A patient in the course of free association had been criticizing me angrily. After a pause, I asked him what he was feeling. He responded, "I feel very guilty." At the time, I was satisfied that I understood the sequence of psychological events. According to the conventional psychoanalytic model, there was a simple cause-and-effect relation between his hostility and guilt; that is, his hostility led directly to guilty feeling. There was no need, according to the theoretical scheme, to interpose any other links in the chain.

But then the patient volunteered the information that while he had been expressing anger-laden criticisms of me, he had also had continual thoughts of a self-critical nature. He described two streams of thought occurring at about the same time: one stream having to do with his hostility and criticisms, which he had expressed in free association, and another that he had not expressed. He then reported the other stream of thoughts: "I said the wrong thing...I shouldn't have said that...I'm wrong to criticize him...I'm bad...He won't like me...I'm bad...I have no excuse for being so mean."

This case presented me with my first clear-cut example of a train of thought running parallel to the reported thought content. I realized that there was a series of thoughts that linked the patient's expression of anger to guilty feelings. Not only was the *intermediate* ideation identifiable, but it directly accounted for the guilty feeling: The patient felt guilty because he had been criticizing himself for his expressions of anger to me.

When I checked subsequently with other patients who had been following the rule of free association for many months or years, I discovered they also had streams of thoughts they had not been reporting. Unlike the first patient, however, many of them were not fully aware of these unreported thoughts until they started to focus on them. Typically, these thoughts differed from the reported ideation in that they appeared to emerge automatically and were extremely rapid. In order to probe into their unexpressed thoughts, I had to guide the patients to be especially attentive to certain ideas and to report them to me. This change of focus was quite revealing, as illustrated in the following case.

A woman who felt continuous unexplained anxiety in the therapy sessions was describing certain sensitive sexual conflicts. Despite mild embarrassment, she verbalized these conflicts freely and without censoring. It was not clear to me why she was experiencing anxiety in each session, so I decided to direct her attention to her thoughts about what she had been saying. Upon my inquiry, she realized that she had been ignoring this stream of ideation. She then reported the following sequence: "I am not expressing myself clearly. . .He is bored with me. . .He probably can't follow what I'm saying. . .This probably sounds foolish to him. . .He will probably try to get rid of me."

As the patient focused on these thoughts and reported them to me, her chronic anxiety during the therapy sessions began to make sense. Her uneasiness had nothing to do with the sexual conflicts she had been describing. But her self-evaluative thoughts and anticipations of my reactions pointed to the essence of her problem. Even though she was actually quite articulate and interesting, she had continual thoughts revolving around the theme of her being inarticulate and boring. After she was able to pinpoint and to correct her unrealistic thoughts, she no longer felt anxious during the therapy sessions.

I noted initially that my patients' automatic thoughts appeared to be of a transference nature: that is, they were concerned with the patient's evaluation of what he was saying or planning to say to me during the session and how he expected me to react to him.[1] Subsequently, the patients recognized they had the same types of thoughts in their interactions with other people. It became increasingly apparent that patients, without realizing it, were constantly communicating with them-

[1] Of course, psychoanalytic writers have always emphasized the importance of the patient's reactions to the analyst. However, they generally enunciated the basic rule without attempting to train the patient to concentrate on his thoughts in the way described in this chapter.

selves outside of therapy as well as in our sessions. By tuning in on the "intercom," as it were, we were able to obtain a more precise definition of the patient's key problems. The woman who thought she was boring me, for instance, recognized similar thoughts in practically all her interpersonal relations.

In order to tap this rich source of information, it was necessary to train patients to observe the stream of unreported thoughts. Since my initial finding had been that these unreported thoughts preceded an emotional state, I instructed the patients, "Whenever you experience an unpleasant feeling or sensation, try to recall what thoughts you had been having prior to this feeling." This instruction helped them to sharpen their awareness of their thoughts, and eventually they were able to identify the thoughts *prior* to experiencing the emotions. Since these thoughts appeared to emerge automatically and extremely rapidly, I labelled them "automatic thoughts." As we shall see in subsequent chapters, the pinpointing of the automatic thoughts provided the raw material for understanding the emotional states and disturbances.

These observations of automatic thoughts presented a dilemma. According to my psychoanalytic training, my patients had been following the basic rule and had expressed the kind of material generally produced by patients in psychoanalysis. This fact was confirmed by my supervisors in the psychoanalytic institute who had reviewed with me the verbatim reports of my patients' free associations. Yet the standard method of emphasizing free association, overcoming censoring, and interpreting resistances, had not (with the exception of the cases described above) yielded the automatic thoughts.

After I considered the problem further, I concluded

that my patients had not really been focusing sharply on the stream of consciousness. They had been presenting material that had to do with current problems, dreams, and memories; or they were presenting narratives of their experiences; or they were jumping from one idea to another in a chain of associations. But they had not concentrated on observing and reporting their thoughts. Ultimately, it became apparent that much of what they reported was based on their conjectures of what they "must be thinking" rather than on sharp focusing on what they were thinking.

Why does conventional free association fail to uncover these automatic thoughts? One possible explanation is that people are accustomed to speaking to themselves in one way and to speaking to others in quite another way. Even though these internal signals exert a powerful influence over him, the patient has a life history of paying no attention to them. He is constantly signaling or communicating with himself as he ceaselessly interprets (or misinterprets) events, monitors his own behavior, makes predictions, and draws generalizations about himself. He is not deterred from reporting these thoughts because of shame or anxiety. Rather, he is either not fully conscious of his automatic thoughts or it does not occur to him that these kinds of thoughts warrant special scrutiny. Only when primed to focus on these thoughts would the patient be likely to report them.

When the patient is more disturbed—as in severe depression—these thoughts are more prominent. In fact, I became more cognizant of their presence when I tried to elicit the thought content from severely depressed patients. I also observed that the automatic thoughts were more compelling in the ideation of obsessional patients.

THE NATURE OF AUTOMATIC THOUGHTS

After my interest in automatic thoughts was aroused, I systematically instructed patients to observe them during free association and to report them to me. I also induced them to record thoughts of this nature that occurred outside of the therapy sessions. In reviewing patients' descriptions of these thoughts, I was struck with the similarities reported by different patients.

From a practical standpoint, the explicit identification of the automatic thoughts relieved me—as well as the patient—of guessing at what he "must be thinking" and made it possible to define with great precision what he was actually thinking. This principle may be illustrated by another case example.

A woman, who was free-associating, was talking about a movie she had seen. In describing the plot of the movie, she reported feeling anxious. When I asked her why she was anxious, she said, "I guess it is because any scenes dealing with aggression probably stir me up." This guess was prompted by her notion derived from psychoanalytic theory that aggression produces anxiety. When I then inquired whether she had been having another chain of thoughts just prior to noticing the anxiety, she responded, "*Now I've got it!* I had the thought that you were critical of me for wasting time by going to the movies. This is what made me nervous."

I noted repeatedly that until a patient had been instructed to focus on the automatic thoughts, they would frequently pass by barely noticed. However, by shifting his attention to these thoughts, the patient could recognize them. As already indicated, the more disturbed a patient was, the more salient were the automatic thoughts. As the patient improved, the automatic thoughts were less obvious; if his condition worsened, the thoughts became more apparent again.

These automatic thoughts reported by numerous patients had a number of characteristics in common. They generally were not vague and unformulated, but were specific and *discrete*. They occurred in a kind of shorthand; that is, only the essential words in a sentence seemed to occur—as in a telegraphic style. Moreover, these thoughts did not arise as a result of deliberation, reasoning, or reflection about an event or topic. There was no logical sequence of steps such as in goal-oriented thinking or problem-solving. The thoughts "just happened," as if by reflex. They seemed to be relatively *autonomous* in that the patient made no effort to initiate them and, especially in the more disturbed cases, they were difficult to "turn off." In view of their involuntary quality they could just as well have been labeled "autonomous thoughts" as automatic thoughts.

In addition, the patient tended to regard these automatic thoughts as *plausible* or reasonable, although they may have seemed far-fetched to somebody else. The patients accepted their validity without question and without testing out their reality or logic. Of course, many of these thoughts were realistic. But the patient often tended to believe the unrealistic thoughts even though he had decided during previous discussions that they were invalid. When he took time out to reflect on their validity or discussed their validity with me, he would conclude they were invalid. Yet, the next time that he had the same automatic thought, he would tend to accept it at face value.

The wording of the thoughts varied according to the circumstances but generally had the same theme. But these were not the typical repetitive thoughts reported by patients with obsessional neurosis. For example, depending upon who was with him, a depressed patient would have the thoughts that his mother was critical of his general behavior or the way he dressed, that his employer disapproved of his performance on the job, that his wife despised his lovemaking, that his therapist devalued his intelligence. These negative thoughts occurred despite the fact that they were contrary to objective evidence. No matter how many times these thoughts were invalidated by external experience, the patient continued to have them—until he recovered from his depression.

I also noted that the content of automatic thoughts, particularly those that were repetitive and seemed to be most powerful, was *idiosyncratic.* They tended to be peculiar not only to the individual patient but to other patients with the same diagnosis. The thoughts were closer to the patient's problems and, therefore, were more useful in psychotherapy than most of what the patient narrated in "free association." As already indicated, these thoughts preceded the arousal of emotion. In the previously cited case, the patient's anxiety was triggered by her automatic thoughts, not by her reflections on the actual content of the movie. Finally, these thoughts generally involved more distortion of reality than did other types of thinking.

It became apparent from my subsequent work with patients that internal signals in a linguistic or visual form play a significant role in behavior. The way a person monitors and instructs himself, praises and criticizes himself, interprets events, and makes predictions not only illuminates normal behavior, but sheds light on the inner workings of the emotional disorders.

SELF-MONITORING AND SELF-INSTRUCTIONS

For a good part of their waking life, people monitor their thoughts, wishes, feelings and actions. Sometimes there is an internal debate as the individual weighs alternatives and courses of action and makes decisions. Plato referred to this phenomenon as an "internal dialogue."

Self-monitoring of behavior may be involved in maladaptive reactions. Overmonitoring can lead to self-consciousness and over-regulation to excessive inhibition. Cautionary signals tend to interfere with spontaneous self-expression. This phenomenon is particularly clear in stage fright, which is generally characterized by an excess of warning signals and inhibiting self-instructions. In obsessional neurosis, the internal debates may paralyze action.

Individuals may also have a *deficit* of self-monitoring of thought and impulse. This deficiency is seen in milder forms in excessive smoking or overeating. The individual blots out awareness of the consequences of his actions. Some food addicts or alcoholics may suspend self-monitoring to the point that they are unaware—or only dimly aware—of starting to eat or drink.

The sequence of scanning the situation, debating, and making decisions leads logically to self-instructions—verbal messages directing behavior. In the most commonplace instances a person gives himself instructions in order to achieve specific, concrete aims. A student reminds himself that it is time to start studying; an entertainer tells himself to pause for applause. Instructing and evaluating oneself also serve broader goals, such as being a good parent, acquiring wealth or power, becoming popular. When a person has a large investment in a particular goal, the relevant instructions take the form of prodding, commanding, and reproaching oneself. Even in the normal state, these proddings and self-instructions can be burdensome.

In a number of clinical conditions, self-instructions may become overmobilized—to the point that a person is constantly driving himself. This quality of being driven by internal prods may be seen among "overachievers" and in the early or mild states of depression. Karen Horney (1950) has described the overly active system of self-commands as "the tyranny of the shoulds." Contradictory "shoulds" may be found in people who are indecisive and in obsessional neurotics.

Another kind of self-instruction revolves around the theme of avoidance or inhibition of action. Such persons react to noxious situations with thoughts of avoidance. When confronted with what appears to be a boring or onerous task, they have the thought, "Don't do it." (Overcoming this resistance may require more willpower than actually doing the task.) Similarly, if people anticipate that a given action might expose them to danger, they may signal themselves to inhibit this action.

Thoughts of escape and avoidance are particularly prominent in the ideation of anxious and depressed patients. The anxious patient perceives danger and, lacking confidence in his capacity to cope with it, experiences wishes and thoughts about escape to safety. The depressed patient regards the usual routines of life as onerous and seeks ways of detaching himself from these burdens or from life itself. He retreats from the perceived unpleasantness into a state of immobility or passivity.

On the other hand, the self-instructions of the angry person take the form of inciting action against the offensive object: "Get even with him"; "Tell him off"; "Don't let him get away with it." The angry, paranoid patient may be propelled into similar action on the basis of illusory offenses.

Self-punishments and self-rewards are related to self-instructions. If the person perceives a deficiency in his behavior or performance, he may barrage himself with regrets and reproaches. He may even make general evaluations of himself as bad, ineffective, or unworthy. The result of such self-reproaches is that he is likely to feel guilty or sad. These reactions, of course, shade into pathological states such as depression in which self-reproaches and self-criticisms are paramount.

The converse of self-punishment or regret is self-reward. When someone is proud of an achievement or receives praise for it, he may think to himself, "You're a great guy. You deserve the best of everything. Happy days are here again!" By the same token, when things go wrong, he is apt to be self-punitive. He thinks, "You look like a fool. You're really not as bright as you thought you were. Everybody considers you a jerk. You really don't have much to offer yourself or anybody else."

ANTICIPATIONS

The role of anticipations in influencing feelings and action is far more dominant than is generally recognized.

The meaning of a person's experiences is very much determined by his expectations of their immediate and ultimate consequences (Kelly, 1955). Whether he is studying, conversing, or working, a person's mood and motivations are elevated by pleasant and dulled by unpleasant expectations.

Anticipations may assume a visual form. A physically ill person may be buoyed by vivid daydreams of regaining his health and pursuing a vigorous life. An anxious person may have visions of disaster as he enters an unknown situation. Depressed patients often have fantasies of failing every task they undertake (Beck, 1970c).

In social situations the individual may attempt to keep score of how other people react to him, and on the basis of his appraisal, he will try to predict what they will think of him. He wonders, "Will they like what I am saying?" "Will they decide I'm a fool?" "Will they praise me?" "Will they mock me?" His natural propensity is to regard any immediate reaction to him as though it will become an enduring attitude. His evaluation of his social image is based largely on what he perceives as the type of impact he makes on others. His notion of his social image may invade his own self-concept. "If I'm not physically attractive, or if I'm a poor conversationalist, people won't like me and I will be worthless."

RULES AND INTERNAL SIGNALS

Consideration of automatic thoughts leads naturally to the question: What general principles shape the content of these internal signals? We know from our own observations that people may behave quite differently in identical circumstances. We find that they interpret the situation differently and evidently issue different "self-instructions." Furthermore, we find that a given person tends to show regularities in his reactions to many situations that are similar in certain crucial respects. His responses may become so predictable that we often attach character attributes to the person: "He is shy and timid." "He is insensitive and aggressive."

These observations of the consistency of responses suggest that each person has a set of general rules that guide how he reacts to specific situations. These rules not only guide his overt actions, but also form the basis for his specific interpretations, his expectancies, and his self-instructions. Furthermore, rules provide the standards by which he judges the efficacy and appropriateness of his actions and evaluates his worth and attractiveness. He uses rules in order to achieve his goals, to protect himself from physical or psychological injury, and to maintain stable relations with others.

The most obvious kinds of rules are standards and regulations. The person uses a kind of mental rule book to guide his actions and evaluate himself and others. He applies the rules in judging whether his own behavior or that of other people is "right" or "wrong." He also uses rules as measuring rods to evaluate the degree of success of a particular performance. By drawing on these standards and principles, he instructs himself (or others) how to behave in a given situation. Afterward, he can evaluate the feedback from his actions, make the necessary corrections, and either praise or criticize himself for his performance.

We use rules not only as a guide for conduct but also to provide a framework for understanding life situations. The rule book contains a coding system used to determine the meanings of stimuli and events. In concrete ways, the rules are used to make arithmetic calculations, to follow a map, to label objects. These rules consist of equations, formulas, and premises that enable the person to order, classify, and synthesize his observations of reality so that he can come to meaningful conclusions.

We also use the code to make sense out of complex situations. When a person tells us something, we not only try to decipher the message, but we extract a highly personal (private) meaning from the communication: We judge whether the other person is offensive to us or whether we are offensive, whether we should strike back or withdraw.

The following example illustrates how the private interpretations of a situation vary according to different rules applied by two individuals. The example also illustrates how different emotions and different forms of behavior are evoked according to which rules are applied.

An instructor, in a casual way, told two students (Miss A and Miss B), who were carrying on a side conversation in his seminar, "If you have anything to say, share it with the rest of us or else be quiet." Miss A responded angrily that she had simply been trying to clarify a point. During the open discussion that followed, she challenged the instructor repeatedly regarding the content of his presentation and expressed sharp criticisms of his point of view. Miss B, who was usually an active participant in the seminar discussions, appeared sad and withdrawn following the instructor's comment, and remained silent for the rest of the class period.

The contrasting responses of these two girls can be understood in terms of different rules they applied in interpreting the situation and then in guiding their overt responses. Miss A interpreted the teacher's remark as "He is trying to control me. He is treating me like a child." Her emotional response was anger. The general rule leading to this interpretation was: "Correction by authority figures = domination and belittling." Her self-instruction was: "Tell him off." The rule behind her retaliation was: "I must get even with people who treat me badly."

Miss B's interpretation: "He has caught me doing something wrong. He will dislike me from now on." Emotion: shame and sadness. Rule: "Correction by authority = exposure and weakness, fault, inferiority. Being corrected = disapproval." Self-instruction: "I should keep my mouth shut." Rule: "If I am quiet, I am less offensive." Also, "Being quiet will show I am sorry for my offensive behavior."

This example illustrates how people operate according to their own specific set of rules. Each girl applied a different rule in assessing the teacher's comment and thus derived a different interpretation. They then applied different rules to yield specific instructions regarding future interactions with the instructor and arrived at opposite conclusions. Their overt behavior simply represented the end product of the internal self-signals.

In summary, these rules may serve as standards to evaluate, steer, or inhibit behaviors; they are applied to others to judge the propriety, justification, and reasonableness of their behavior. By applying these rules, standards, or principles, the individual evaluates the significance of other peoples' actions and interprets how they regard his actions.

How do these rules originate? We know that people speak grammatically before they are taught the formal rules of grammar. They are not told explicitly in early childhood that they should follow a particular sequence of subject-verb-object (for example, "I want my bottle"). They derive the general rules from concrete experiehces. They also behave in a socialized fashion before general rules of conduct are articulated to them. Inasmuch as rules are part of the social heritage, they are probably absorbed to a large extent through observations of other people as well as from personal experiences. It is fairly easy to see how a general rule ("Be polite" or "Stick up for your rights") is applied to a specific situation to produce specific behavior. Similarly, we can see how a rule determines the interpretation of the situation.

The operation of the rules can be compared to the kind of syllogisms discussed by logicians. For example, Miss A and Miss B have as a major premise, the rule: "All corrections by a person in authority are criticisms." The minor premise is "The teacher is correcting me." "Therefore," they conclude, "the teacher is criticizing me." The person does not actually state the initial premise to himself. The premise is already part of his cognitive organization just as are the rules for constructing sentences or the rules for distinguishing between animals and plants. Depending on the circumstances, the person may or may not have a concrete thought about the special case. In any event, he is aware of the conclusion. The conclusion may assume a central position or may be fleeting like the automatic thoughts previously described.

The rules and the syllogisms based on the rules are of particular interest to the clinician because they help to explain unpredictable, illogical behavior and abnormal emotional responses. In Chapter 4, we shall see that when the rules are discordant with reality or are applied excessively or arbitrarily, they are likely to produce psychological or interpersonal problems.

CHAPTER 3

Meaning and Emotions

Men are not moved by things but the views which they take of them.—Epictetus

THE MEANING OF MEANING

Why do so many students of human nature and its aberrations turn away from conscious meanings? Meaning provides the richness of life; it transforms a simple event into an experience. Yet, contemporary systems of psychology and psychiatry either completely disregard meanings or go to extremes in seeking esoteric ones. Behaviorism detours around thoughts and "mentalistic concepts." Classical psychoanalysis, dissatisfied with "superficial" meanings, takes flight into an elaborate infrastructure of symbolic meanings that are contrary to common-sense meanings of an event.

Despite their many differences, behaviorists and psychoanalysts are similar in their reluctance to accept a patient's description of his psychological processes at face value; both schools are skeptical of "common-sense" explanations of behavior. The behaviorists dismiss people's reports of their "subjective" experience as unreliable because the experiences cannot be verified by other observers. Psychoanalysts assume conscious ideation is simply a product of unconscious forces which work to disguise the "real meaning" of events. Neuropsychiatrists are content with notions such as, "under every twisted thought is a twisted molecule." The psychological meaning of the aberration does not interest them.

In contrast to the "hard-headed" behaviorist and neuropsychiatric attitudes and the abstract classical psychoanalytic position, the cognitive approach is concerned with conscious meanings as well as external events. The person's reports of his ideas, feelings, and wishes provide the raw material for the cognitive model. Furthermore, his various interpretations of events are accepted as basic, rock-bottom data—not as a superficial screen over "deeper" meanings such as the psychoanalysts postulate. At times, it may be necessary to sift the automatic thoughts and other introspective data to delineate the intricate pattern of meanings and connotations. The formulation is then "tried on for size" and may have to be reworked until the patient determines that it fits his particular construction of reality.

To understand the emotional reactions to an event, it is necessary to make a distinction between the dictionary or "public" meaning of an occurrence and its personal or private meaning. The public meaning is the formal, objective definition of the event—devoid of personal significance or connotation. A boy is teased by his friends: The objective meaning of the event is simply that they are goading him. The personal meaning for the boy who is teased is more complex, for example, "They don't like me" or "I am a weakling." Although he is aware of this special meaning, he generally keeps it to himself because he knows that if he admits his private reactions openly, his friends will probably tease him even more. A girl who receives the best grade in her class may think, "This shows I am better than the other students," but she is not likely to express this special meaning lest she antagonize her classmates. Special meanings are evoked when an event touches on an important part of a person's life, such as acceptance by peers, but they frequently remain private and unexpressed.

Private meanings are often unrealistic because the person does not have the opportunity to check their authenticity. In fact, when patients reveal such meanings to their psychotherapist, this is frequently the first chance they have had to examine these hidden meanings and to test their validity. A successful salesman in his mid-fifties became intensely anxious when told he must enter a hospital for treatment of pneumonia. Although he acknowledged the usual conception of a hospital as a place where illness is treated, his private notion (as revealed by his automatic thoughts) centered on anticipations of being anesthetized, cut up, carted off to a morgue. His anxiety was produced by the personal meaning—not by the socially accepted definition of a hospital.

At times we find that a person's reactions to an event are completely inappropriate or so excessive as to seem abnormal. When we question him, we often find that he has misinterpreted the situation. His misinterpretation comprises a web of incorrect meanings he has attached to the situation. Intepretations that consistently depart from reality (and are not simply based on incorrect information) can be justifiably labeled as deviant. As we shall see, the deviant meanings constitute the cognitive distortions that form the core of emotional disorders.

A person may have to concentrate on his stream of thoughts or images at the time of an event in order to pinpoint its personal meaning. For example, a medical student experiencing horror at seeing a patient bleeding during an operation was unable initially to understand his exaggerated reaction. However, after prodding his memory, he recalled that, at the time, he had experienced a visual image of *himself* bleeding and also remembered having had the thought, "This could happen to me!" The fantasy and thought rather than the sight of the patient were the key factor in evoking horror. Observing the same sight during subsequent operations no longer produced either the unpleasant feeling or the fantasy.

Meanings, significances, and imagery comprise what has been called "internal reality." Psychoanalysts have made Herculean efforts to explore it, but, reluctant to accept patients' reports at face value, have recast the ideational material into theory-derived constructs. Even when meanings are elusive, however, careful introspection and reporting of internal experiences help to expand a person's awareness to encompass a continuous flow of images and thoughts. The nature of this cognitive flow was described in Chapter 2.

THE ROUTE TO THE EMOTIONS

We have noted that common-sense observations and generalizations form the groundwork for the physical sciences. These generalizations are derived from establishing a causal relation between events and physical phenomena: The support is removed from an object and it falls. Similar kinds of relations may be demonstrated in developing a scientific approach to psychological phenomena. However, in contrast to the early stages in physical sciences, the most significant data are subjective and intrapsychic rather than objective and external. Only the person who actually experiences the emotion, idea, and image can make and report his introspective observations. Tentative relations among these psychological experiences established for a given person may be confirmed by comparing them with relevant reports from other persons. In this way, generalizations are gradually developed. In addition, the sequence from external, objective events to specific ideas, to emotional reaction may be traced in order to determine consistencies as well as differences among individuals.

Consider the following example of how a specific external event evokes meaning for different people. A teacher remarked to her class that Tony, a bright student, received a low grade on a test. One student was pleased—he thought, "This shows I'm smarter than Tony." Tony's best friend felt sad (as did Tony): He shared Tony's loss. Another student was frightened: "If Tony did poorly, I may have done poorly also." Still another student became incensed at the teacher: "She probably marked unfairly if she gave Tony a low grade." By being "unfair" to one student, she had violated a cardinal rule and, therefore, she could be unfair to any student. Finally, a visiting student had no emotional response at all: Tony's grade had no special meaning for him.

This example demonstrates an essential relation: The specific content of the interpretation of an event leads to a specific emotional response. Further, based on examination of numerous similar examples, we can generalize that, depending on the kind of interpretation a person makes, he will feel glad, sad, scared, or angry—or he may have no particular emotional reaction at all.

The diverse personal meanings of an event not only account for the variety of emotional responses to the same situation but have direct application to understanding emotional problems. A person who attaches an unrealistic or extravagant meaning to an event is likely to experience an inappropriate or excessive emotional response. A man lying in bed who imagines that each noise is a burglar breaking into the house will feel excessive anxiety. If he consistently interprets innocuous stimuli as danger signals, he may develop an anxiety neurosis.

The thesis that the special meaning of an event determines the emotional response forms the core of the cognitive model of emotions and emotional disorders: The meaning is encased in a cognition—a thought or an image. Sometimes the cognition may consist simply of a connotation or value judgment such as "awful" or "wonderful." It is a commonplace observation that a particular emotion may have no connection to the external circumstances at the time. If we are daydreaming or ruminating, our emotion is generated by the content of the reverie or ideas (rather than by an external stimulus). Finally, if we distort a situation grossly, our emotional response is consistent with the distortion rather than with the factual aspects of the situation.

The cognitive model of emotions is derived, initially, from reports of introspective observations of thoughts and feelings. Second, the relation of thought to feeling is determined. Third, generalizations are made regarding what kinds of thoughts (or meanings) lead to which emotions.

Other theories of emotions have ignored or have not

adequately used people's reports of their thinking and feeling. Classical behaviorism uses a stimulus-response model to explain emotional reactions. It proposes a simpler route by which an external event leads directly to an emotional response—without interposing thinking or meaning between stimulus and response. According to behavioral theory, the sequence between stimulus and response has been established as the result of previous conditioning; hence, this formulation is often referred to as the conditioning model.

The classical psychoanalytic model of emotions is far more complex. Reduced to simple terms, the sequence is as follows: A stimulus or event occurs and arouses an unconscious wish or impulse. Since the wish is generally unacceptable to the person, its incipient emergence into consciousness poses an internal threat. If he is unable to ward off the taboo impulse through the use of a defense mechanism, he experiences anxiety or guilt. For example, according to Freud's concept of the Oedipus complex, a young boy reacts to the sight of his mother (the stimulus) with an unconscious sexual impulse directed toward her. If the wish threatens to break into consciousness, the boy feels anxious because of possible punishment from his rival—the father.[1]

The behavioral and psychoanalytic models are similar in that they minimize the importance of meanings that are accessible to introspective observation and report. The behaviorists reject meaning totally and the psychoanalysts emphasize unconscious meanings. The

[1] The child's stream of ideas is less esoteric. If questioned about his thoughts and feelings, he is likely to state that the sight of his mother stirs up a rather prosaic fear—such as the fear of being punished for making a mess, for having hit a younger sibling, or for having done poorly in school.

models differ in the location of the controlling stimulus: According to the conditioning model, it is external; according to the psychoanalytic model, it is internal but unconscious (See Figure 1).

The psychoanalytic and behavioral models skirt the common conceptions of why a person becomes sad, glad, afraid, or angry. The cognitive approach, however, brings the whole matter of arousal of emotion back within the range of common-sense observation. By sorting out the specific meanings of events, this approach draws together many diverse or dissimilar situations that lead to the same emotional response. Although at times the specific conditions for the arousal of a particular emotion may seem too obvious to warrant fine-grained analysis, they are crucial to the development of the generalizations. These generalizations, in turn, serve as the basis for understanding emotional disorders such as depression, mania, anxiety neurosis, and paranoid states.

THE PERSONAL DOMAIN

A man was shown a picture of a coat of arms by a friend. He was indifferent to it until he was persuaded that it was actually a picture of his own family's coat of arms. From then on, he prized the picture, was excited in showing it to other people, and was hurt when they seemed uninterested. He reacted to the illustration on the piece of paper as though it were an extension of himself.

This incident illustrates how a person attaches special meanings to, and is moved by, objects that he judges to be of particular relevance to him. The objects—tangible and intangible—in which he has such an involvement constitute his personal domain. At the center of the

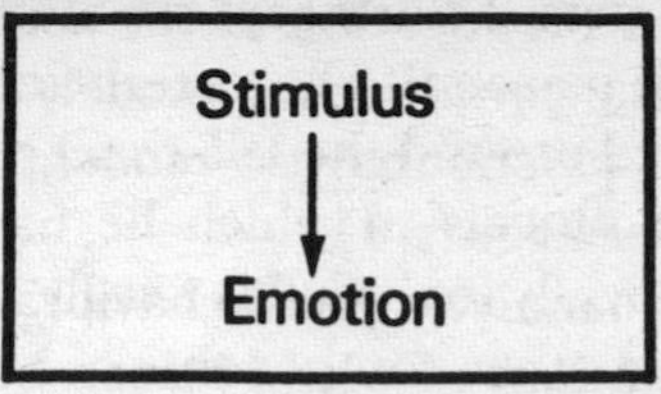

Conditioning Model

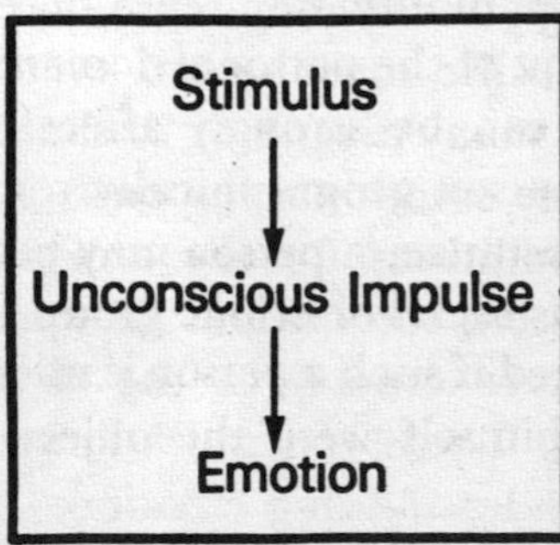

Psychoanalytic Model

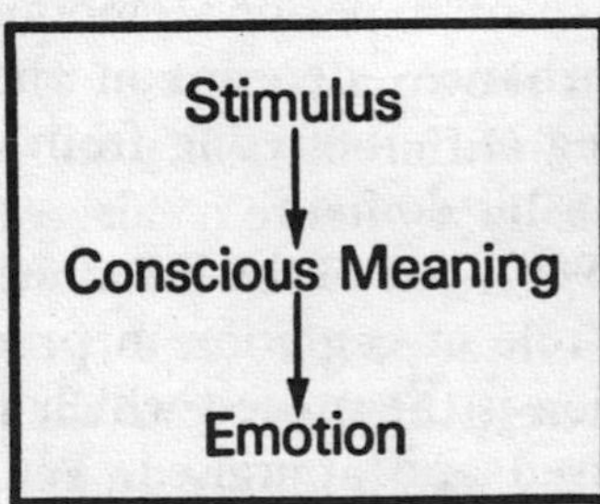

Cognitive Model

FIGURE 1

THINKING AND EMOTION

domain is the person's concept of himself, his physical attributes and personal characteristics, his goals and values. Clustered around the self-concept are the animate and inanimate objects in which he has an investment. The objects typically include his family, friends, material possessions. The other components of his domain vary in degree of abstractness: from his school, social group, and nationality to intangible values or ideals concerning freedom, justice, morality.

The concept of the personal domain helps to explain how a person can be strongly affected even when an institution or person geographically remote from him is involved. For instance, a person may become euphoric if a member of his racial or ethnic group is honored, or he may feel outraged if such a person is mistreated. He reacts as though he himself were the object of good or bad treatment.

As we analyze the circumstances relevant to the emotions and the emotional disorders, the importance of the concept of the personal domain will become apparent. The nature of a person's emotional response—or emotional disturbance—depends on whether he perceives events as adding to, subtracting from, endangering, or impinging upon his domain.

Arnold (1960), one of the first theorists to elaborate on the central role of cognition in producing emotions, asserts, "Emotion is the process which starts when something is perceived and appraised. We decide that it is good or bad for us." Depending on whether someone appraises a stimulus as beneficial or detrimental to his personal domain, he experiences a "positive" or "negative" reaction. "Something good for me" leads to emotions such as joy, pleasure, happiness. Something appraised as bad induces sadness, anxiety, or anger.

Although Arnold, experimental psychologists such as Richard Lazarus (1966), and clinicians such as Albert Ellis (1962), have clearly marked the route between thinking and emotion, they have not delineated the particular kinds of appraisals that lead to specific emotions. In fact, the vast literature in personality and social psychology hardly touches on the question of what ideational content in response to a noxious stimulus or a threat produces, respectively, sadness, anxiety, or anger. Granted that the initial appraisal may be a global "bad for me," the individual's unique interpretation of the noxious stimulus determines his emotional response.

SADNESS

Sadness is not only a ubiquitous human experience, but at times, is the most puzzling. How often have we heard a child or even an adult say, "I'm sad but I don't know why!" The sad feeling is often contrary to the apparent life situation. A person "who has everything" may feel sad and another person "who has nothing" may be content and even happy.

Consider some typical instances of paradoxical sadness. (1) A salesman received news that he was promoted to a higher position in his business organization. To his surprise his reaction was sadness rather than joy. (2) A mother felt unhappy when her long-time ambition was fulfilled: Her daughter married a very suitable man. (3) A college graduate attended a class reunion he had eagerly anticipated for many years. As he mingled with his old friends he felt a pall of gloom descend over him. (4) After moving into his "dream house," a middle-aged man began to feel sad.

Can any common meaning be wrung from these

experiences? The information supplied by each person provides a plausible explanation for his sad reaction. The salesman became disheartened when he thought, "I will be moving far away. I don't have any friends there." The mother managed to identify the automatic thought that precipitated the gloom: "I have lost my baby." The college alumnus experienced a low mood as he began comparing himself unfavorably with his friends and judging himself a failure. The new homeowner became sad as he thought about the "stark reality" of how much money his house had cost him.

Although each of these people had in actuality added to his domain by attaining a long-cherished goal, his dominant interpretation was the opposite: *Something of value has been lost.*

The special meaning of a particular loss determines whether a person will feel sad: namely, if he conceives of the loss as subtracting from his domain in some significant way. For example, a millionnaire who accidentally loses a few dollars might be indifferent to this loss because it doesn't perceptibly affect his financial worth; however, he might become sad if he lost the same amount of money on a bet, because then the loss would have negative connotations regarding his judgment or luck. Similarly, a criticism from a disoriented patient may not hurt a psychiatrist if he does not value the patient's judgment. The same criticism by a colleague may substantially lower the psychiatrist's self-esteem. If the person does not value an attribute, he is not disturbed at its removal from his domain. The loss of a wart is likely to produce satisfaction, but the loss of hair, sadness.

It is easy to observe how many life situations can be interpreted as a loss or can lead to a reduced valuation of the domain. The different kinds of events that may lead to sadness can be readily categorized:

1. Loss of a tangible object that is considered a source of gratification or is valued for some other reason.

2. An intangible loss such as the diminished self-esteem produced by an insult or disparagement.

3. A reversal in the value of a component of the domain; for example, what was regarded as an asset is now judged negatively.

4. A discrepancy between what is expected and what is actually received, i.e., a disappointment.

5. A fantasy or expectation of a future loss: The individual tends to live through the anticipated loss as though it were happening *right now,* and so he experiences the sadness before the loss actually occurs.

6. Hypothetical loss: No loss has occurred but it "could" happen.

7. Pseudo loss: The person incorrectly perceives an event as subtracting from his domain.

Actual loss may refer to deprivation of something tangible and definable, such as money. An intangible loss, such as the loss of another person's affection, may produce a sad feeling like that produced by the loss of a tangible object. Similarly, a reversal in a person's evaluation of an attribute may trigger sadness; for example, a person who previously regarded himself as humorous may decide that people regard him simply as a buffoon.

The intensity of the sense of loss is proportional to the amount of depreciation in the value of the attribute rather than its "absolute value." A girl, for example, who had previously regarded herself as beautiful, determined that people considered her merely pretty: Her sense of loss and sadness corresponds to the degree she considered herself less desirable than previously. Similarly, a parent who had regarded his child as an exceptional student felt sad upon learning that the child was simply above average.

The ideation involved in unfulfilled expectations and disappointment also incorporates the theme of loss and triggers sadness. When a person expects to receive an honor, prize, or salary raise, he immediately takes partial title to it, as it were. While the object occupies its fantasied place in his domain, he generally experiences some gratification. If he does not receive the expected object, he may experience as much sadness as though he had actually received and then lost it. Intense disappointment is experienced even though the expectation was highly unrealistic.

Many people "live the future in the present" and experience an anticipated loss as actual. A woman, when informed that her husband would be leaving in a few months for a brief business trip, felt as sad as she did when he actually left. When she thought ahead to the time when her children would grow up and leave the house, she was brought to tears.

When a possible loss is treated as though it were an actual deprivation, it is labeled a hypothetical loss. A woman would feel sad, for instance, whenever her husband talked to another woman. She would think, "It's possible that he may be falling in love with her."

Invalid "bookkeeping" is an example of a pseudo loss: A man experienced a sense of loss whenever he spent money to acquire something of value—until he was helped to realize that the expense was more than balanced by the acquisition.

EUPHORIA AND EXCITATION

Just as common-sense observation links sadness to loss, the necessary condition for euphoria or excitation is the perception or expectation of gain. The person increases his evaluation of his domain. The boundaries of the domain may be expanded, for example, by adding new friends, by acquiring new tangible objects, or by attaining a goal. A woman may rate her social abilities more highly after her first successful dinner party; a man may like a new suit more after he has been complimented on it.

Not only does a positive appraisal, which leads to self-enhancement, produce feelings of euphoria but *anticipation* of future pleasure or enhancements may also lead to immediate pleasure. In fact, this kind of anticipatory thinking can have an escalating effect. For example, a man noted a description of some of his professional work in a newspaper article, and his first thought was that his work (actually *he*) was very important to warrant so much publicity. This idea produced a noticeable elevation in his mood. He then thought of all the people who would see this article, and his euphoria increased markedly. Next, he fantasied receiving greater publicity and becoming increasingly famous. With each successive broadening of his expectations, there was a corresponding boost in his mood.

Whether or not the person experiences pleasure depends on the meaning attached to a particular situation or object. A young man observed that a girl was watching him. He thought, "Nancy likes me." He then generalized this conclusion to: "Because she likes me, her friends will like me." Then: "I guess I'm pretty popular. People in general like me." As he expanded his positive evaluations, he felt a corresponding elevation of mood.

It is not necessary to have a pre-existing "need" or "drive" fulfilled in order to experience pleasure. Any event—or idea—that represents a meaningful addition is sufficient to produce pleasure. A person, for instance, may unexpectedly receive a gift without ever having wanted it and may, nonetheless, experience pleasure. However, once he has felt pleasure, *then* the person may develop an active desire for more of the pleasure-producing object. A taste of fame may make a person hungry for more in order to maintain his new self-evaluation.

Thus, an increase in self-evaluation may have a substantial effect on motivation. Receiving a reward can result in a generalized increase in the expectation of rewards, and consequently energize the person to work more productively. This principle is particularly useful in helping depressed patients overcome their inertia.

Feedback mechanisms may play a role in escalating the response to gains. The subjective experience of euphoria after a self-enhancing event may be interpreted as further evidence that the event is a "good thing." This positive appraisal may stimulate further desires for the pleasure-inducing object or circumstances.

ANXIETY

It is a commonplace observation that when someone considers himself in imminent danger he is likely to feel anxious. Threats of physical harm, serious illness, economic disaster, or social rejection quickly come to mind as typical anxiety-producing situations. Moreover, we can observe that a threat (real or imaginary) to the safety, health, or psychological state of any other person within his personal domain may also produce anxiety. A person may also become anxious if he perceives a danger to some institution or principle he values.

The prospect of losing some important object, animate or inanimate, is another common kind of threat to the personal domain. A person may become anxious when threatened with losing money or material possessions. Anxiety may also be induced by the anticipated loss of a friend or relative through geographical separation, sickness, or death of the other person. Anxiety in response to psychosocial threats (such as anticipation of criticism, humiliation, or desertion) has the same quality as distress over threats of physical harm or illness.

We label anticipation of damage fear, and the unpleasant emotional reaction anxiety.[2] If a person feels confident in his ability to cope with or repel the threat, anxiety is minimized. It is increased when he considers the potential damage to his domain as imminent, highly probable, and highly destructive. Anxiety may be further increased by uncertainty with regard to when the harm may occur.

In identifying a situation as dangerous, one must make a series of almost simultaneous judgments. The initial judgment, which Richard Lazarus (1966) terms "primary appraisal," identifies the situation as a threat and assesses the probability, imminence, and degree of the potential harm. Next comes secondary appraisal—an estimate of one's "counter-harm" resources; that is, ability to neutralize or cope with the danger. The ratio

[2] The distinction between fear and anxiety will be elaborated in Chapter 6.

between the negative factors in the primary appraisal and the positive factors in the secondary appraisal constitutes the perceived risk. The latter in turn, determines the intensity of anxiety.

The importance of meaning in the arousal is illustrated by the large variety of situations that produce this emotional response and in the degree to which it occurs in different individuals in the same situation. We are familiar with the fact that someone who is highly sensitive to social disapproval may become alarmed if placed in a situation in which his weaknesses could be exposed; for example, he may consider having to speak before an audience as a potential catastrophe. Another person will experience minimal or no anxiety in such a situation because he attaches a different meaning to other people's possible evaluations of him.

Similarly, unusual anxiety reactions to situations or objects that are generally considered safe are found to be related to private, idiosyncratic meanings. A healthy woman, for instance, experienced anxiety whenever she became short of breath following exertion because she thought she was having a heart attack. A man felt anxious whenever he was on a bridge because as he crossed over he would have a visual image of the bridge collapsing. Later we shall consider other illustrations of the crucial role of meaning in pathological states of anxiety.

ANGER

One of the examples occasionally cited as the prototype of anger is the reaction of a primitive organism to destroy or repel a noxious agent. This analogy illuminates one basic pattern in humans: When a person is attacked (physically or verbally), he may become angry and counterattack.

Although the formula, "attack leads to anger," fits some of the most obvious conditions for generation of anger, it does not always apply. We know of instances in which an attacked person has felt paralyzed with anxiety or has become sad after being defeated in a physical battle. Other mammals, such as chimpanzees and dogs, respond to attack with reactions that seem to resemble human anxiety or depression. Cannon (1915) describes reactions to attack in terms of a fight-or-flight pattern, corresponding roughly to anger or anxiety. His formula, however, does not account for a depressive response, nor does it specify the reasons for individual differences.

Another familiar situation that often produces anger is the frustration of a wish or drive. This common observation, was expanded by Dollard et al. (1939) into a broad theory (the frustration-aggression hypothesis), proposing to account for the spectrum of aggressive and hostile behavior. When subjected to critical analysis, however, it becomes apparent that their concept encompasses only a limited range of anger-producing situations. Furthermore, by overlooking the *meaning* of frustration under varying circumstances, the authors include instances of frustration that do not produce anger. As pointed out by Ellis (1962), and demonstrated experimentally by Pastore (1950, 1952), people are unlikely to respond with anger if they judge the frustrating agent to be justified, nonarbitrary or reasonable. A husband who generally becomes angry if his dinner is not ready when he comes home will not be annoyed if he discovers his wife was too sick to prepare the meal.

If we reflect on the kinds of situations that can

produce anger, ranging from mild irritation to extreme fury, we can probably think of an almost endless variety. We would be hard-put to consider the different kinds of anger-producing situations as all related in some way. Nonetheless, by singling out the central features of these situations, it is possible to expose the bonds of kinship.

TRANSGRESSIONS—INTENTIONAL AND UNINTENTIONAL

Consider these examples from the broad spectrum of everyday situations that often produce anger: (1) An adult is pelted with stones by a gang of adolescents. (2) A student is singled out for reprimand by his teacher for whispering with several other students during class. (3) A theater-goer's attempt to purchase a ticket is thwarted by somebody pushing ahead of him in line at the box office. (4) A woman is jilted by her lover. (5) A child is told by his parent that he must share his toys with a sibling. (6) A member of a committee attempting to introduce a new policy is opposed by other committeemen.

At least one common thread runs through each of these confrontations. The main character (or protagonist) is subjected to an unpleasant experience (the offense) by one or more adversaries: He is the object of *deliberate* physical attack, criticism, coercion, thwarting, rejection, deprivation, or opposition. These situations are noxious because they encroach on the protagonist's safety, self-esteem, or desires; they are perceived as a deliberate, direct impingement on his domain. Even when the offense is not motivated by malice, it may be perceived as such by the protagonist.

Another group of anger-producing situations is composed of commands and restrictions which the individual interprets as encroaching on his rights. A restriction by a person in authority may make an individual angry though he had no prior desire to engage in the forbidden activity. His "rights" may include not only autonomy, freedom of action, and freedom of expression, but also expectations of respect, courtesy, consideration, and loyalty from other people. Social or professional status may prompt the expectation of special privileges and may cause offense if they are not accorded, or anger if a person of lower status tries to claim privileges to which he is not "entitled."

INDIRECT TRANSGRESSIONS

Still another type of interaction accounts for many of the angry responses we experience ourselves or may observe in others. The following situations do not appear at first glance to represent a direct assault on the domain; yet, they may produce anger: (1) A host feels annoyed at a guest for showing off his knowledge at a dinner party. (2) A clerical worker is irritated at a friend's stories of his success in business. (3) A young man is furious with his girl friend for chatting in an animated way with another man. (4) A student who received an outstanding grade becomes annoyed at his professor when he learns the professor gave the same grade to a fellow student. (5) A husband is infuriated because his wife gives him only a mild compliment for what he considers a major business triumph.

On analyzing these situations, we can understand why they are regarded as noxious: The meaning of each is an assault on the self-esteem of the protagonist. The behavior of the offender *indirectly* exposes the protagonist to self-devaluation. The first group of incidents are examples of jealousy or envy. The attention-getters are offensive because they threaten to dim the image of the protagonist: "He is getting all the recognition and I'm not getting any," "He is making a better impression than I," "He is more successful than I." Such comparisons lead the protagonist to question his own importance. The student's enhanced self-esteem for receiving an outstanding grade is diminished when he loses the exclusiveness of his claim to excellence. The husband is annoyed at his wife's lukewarm response because it seems to devalue his achievement.

Since the "offenses" represent a kind of loss, why does the protagonist feel angry rather than sad? We find that he experiences anger as long as he is able to ward off his devaluation by focusing on negative attributes of the offender: He is a "show-off," undeserving, empty-headed, unfair. If, however, the protagonist accepts the imagined loss of status as reasonable, just, or fair, then he feels sad. If he fluctuates between blaming the offender and regretting his loss, his mood oscillates between anger and sadness.

HYPOTHETICAL TRANSGRESSIONS

We can think of other instances in which neither a direct nor an indirect transgression seems to account for an angry reaction: (1) A pedestrian becomes angry at seeing a motorist drive through a stop signal. (2) A parent is incensed at his child for not showing "good table manners." (3) A wealthy man is infuriated at being approached for a charitable contribution. (4) A man devoted to the principle of law and order becomes enraged at hearing of a crime committed thousands of miles away.

None of these episodes produces an obvious infringement on the individual's domain; yet, he may react as strongly as he would to a direct assault. He may readily acknowledge that he was in no way personally damaged by the event. If this is correct, then why is he angered? The common denominator in each of these incidents is that the offender has violated a rule regarded as important to the offended. Because this violation leads the protagonist to regard himself as vulnerable, it represents a potential or hypothetical transgression.

The pedestrian explains his anger at the speeding motorist: "I *could have been* walking across the street at that time" (or might have crossed at some future time when the motorist was speeding through). The parent is annoyed with her child because she conjectures that, if an outsider were present, he might judge her to be a bad mother for rearing "an ill-mannered child." The wealthy man is incensed because he speculates, "If I had to give money to every charity, I would go broke."

In hypothetical attacks, the notion that it *could* happen carries almost as much weight as if it *did* happen. The hypothetical infringements, although subtle, account for a large proportion of the discord in human relations. As we proceed, we shall see that these offenses consist largely of the violation of some generally accepted rules of proper behavior or, in some instances, certain idiosyncratic rules and standards.

The imposition of a value judgment on other people's behavior points to the existence of an implicit code of laws, rules, principles, and standards. These rules seem to be applied as though they serve to protect the protagonist from physical or psychological harm even though his person and his domain are in no way involved in an interaction with the offender. Thus, the pedestrian, although not actually endangered, becomes furious at the motorist because violation of the law might affect his future safety.

The principles of fair play, justice, and reasonableness constitute a kind of outer wall or defense of the domain. Arbitrary, unfair, unjust acts arouse anger (even when not directed against a particular person) because they are regarded as a threat to the protective wall.

Other customs affecting human interactions are heavily invested with importance. Diagnostic clues of the violation of such conventions are found in angry complaints such as: "They have no right to act that way." "He should not have done that." "Those people should behave better." "It's the principle of the thing."

A middle-aged business executive becomes irritated by a host of behavior patterns in other persons such as their being "loud-mouthed," aggressive, careless, or unkempt. On being questioned, he readily admits that he has not personally experienced any injury or loss from this behavior. He protests nonetheless that such behavior is "wrong" or "bad" and that the offender should be punished in some way: "Those hippies have no business wearing their hair so long and being so dirty. They should be locked up."

Acceptable forms of behavior constitute a moral code that is embedded in the domain. *A breach of the code produces the same reaction as an attack.* The personal code varies widely within a cultural group, and may be idiosyncratic. Anger produced by violation of such codes may seem inappropriate and unhealthy to others, but it seems appropriate to the individual, who has his own standards of right and wrong. A violation of his personal standards is regarded as an attack on his domain.

Social conventions appear to play a greater role than is generally recognized in specifying the conditions under which anger is considered justified, expected, or even demanded, but also set the limits beyond which anger is deemed excessive or inappropriate. Such limits are implied in statements such as "You're over-reacting," or "Why the temper tantrum?" We have probably all encountered situations that made us angry but did not affect a friend, and vice versa. Similarly, when we have reacted with equanimity to a noxious situation, we may have been told, "You should have gotten angry," or "I would have told him off!" When a person exhibits a strong outburst of anger over what is generally regarded as a trivial incident, we may suspect that the situation has a special idiosyncratic meaning for him.

We can now summarize the kinds of situations that commonly lead to anger: (1) direct and intentional attack; (2) direct, unintentional attack; (3) violation of laws, standards, social mores: hypothetical threats, substandard behavior, breach of idiosyncratic moral code. The common factor for arousal of anger is the individual's appraisal of an assault on his domain, including his values, moral code, and protective rules. This factor, while a necessary condition, is not sufficient in itself to arouse anger. In order to provoke anger, other specific conditions must be present. First, the individual must take the infringement seriously and label it negatively. A small child throwing snowballs at his parent is likely to provoke amusement rather than anger. Second, the individual must not consider the noxious situation an immediate or continuing danger. If he is concerned primarily with his own safety, he will be more anxious than angry. Third, the individual must focus primarily on the wrongfulness of the offense and the offender rather than on any injury he may have sustained.

The sequence of psychological reactions leading to anger may be compared with the steps in the production of anxiety. The individual makes a primary appraisal in recognizing and labeling the noxious stimulus. Concomitantly, he assesses his ability to sustain, neutralize, or repel the impact of the noxious stimulus (secondary appraisal). In the following example, the protagonist fluctuated between anger and anxiety as his confidence in his ability to repel the noxious stimulus increased and faded.

A college student was blocked in traffic by a slowly moving car. He became very angry because he was both inconvenienced and offended by the other driver's disregard for an accepted rule of driving. He sounded his horn repeatedly and swore at the driver—he regarded himself as strong enough to cope with possible retaliation which, in any event, he considered unlikely. To his surprise, the other driver got out of his car. The student was angered even further at such pugnacity. When it became plain that the second driver was huge and menacing, the student became anxious and drove off quickly. When he was a safe distance away, the student felt another wave of anger as he reflected, "The big bully—trying to push me around."

This example illustrates that when a person is not concerned about his safety, he is prone to experience anger toward the offending agent. When he focuses primarily on imminent danger, his anger is replaced by anxiety.

Analogous fluctuations between anger and sadness

were experienced by a man whose wife had reprimanded him severely. One moment he would think about how unjust she was to criticize him, and he would feel angry at her. Then, he would shift to the idea that he had lost her affection, and would feel sad. All day the focus of his thinking alternated between blaming his wife and being deprived of love, with corresponding oscillations between anger and sadness.

The degree of anger is generally proportional to how unreasonable, arbitrary, or improper the offense seems to the protagonist. These characteristics are of extreme importance in understanding excessive reactions to what may seem to be trivial offenses.

The conditions that *accentuate anger* after an offense has occurred may be summarized as follows: (1) offense perceived as intentional; (2) offense perceived as malicious; (3) offense perceived as unjustified, unfair, unreasonable; (4) offender perceived as undesirable person; (5) possibility of blaming or disqualifying offender.

Converse conditions tend to reduce the anger, e.g., the offense is perceived as "accidental," "well-intentioned," or "justified." Other mitigating factors are the protagonist's view of the offender "as a nice guy" or his belief that he himself was at fault.

DISTINGUISHING AMONG AROUSAL OF SADNESS, ANGER, AND ANXIETY

Everyday observation indicates that the same external conditions may produce sadness in one person, anxiety in another, and anger in a third. Moreover, circumstances that seem basically alike may make someone sad at one time, anxious at another time, and angry a third time. If we know the meanings attached to the event, we can generally predict which emotion will be aroused. Paramount meanings are determined by the person's habitual patterns of conceptualizing particular kinds of life situations and also by his psychological state at the time the situation occurs. If his main concern is with danger, he feels anxious; if he is preoccupied with loss, he feels sad; if he focuses on the unacceptable behavior of the offender, he feels angry. The necessary and sufficient conditions for the arousal of each emotion may be demonstrated by pinpointing how similar conditions may produce different emotions.

SADNESS VERSUS ANGER

Downgrading (as by insult or criticism) may produce either sadness or anger. If one accepts the validity of the insult sufficiently to lower his evaluation of himself, then he feels sad. Similarly, even when he considers an insult invalid, he may feel sad provided he considers merely being insulted a bad reflection on him. If the criticism or insult is perceived as unwarranted, unacceptable, or unjust, he is likely to experience anger.

The person may realize that if he accepts the validity of the "criticism," he may feel sad or guilty. However, if he can discredit the criticism by disqualifying his critic, he is likely to experience anger instead of sadness.

SADNESS VERSUS ANXIETY

A person is likely to feel sad rather than anxious when the loss has already occurred or when the domain has been devalued in expectation of a loss. He will experience anxiety as long as he regards himself as still intact and the loss or other injury as only imminent. An example of the production of sadness rather than anxiety in anticipation of a noxious event is the knowledge of some future loss—be it an important person, job, or status. Sadness results if the projected loss is experienced in the present rather than in the future, that is, when the person makes the subtraction from his domain before the actual loss occurs.

ANXIETY VERSUS ANGER

For the arousal of anxiety, the salient feature is *danger:* The person is concerned primarily with the possibility of being hurt and with his perceived lack of coping devices to deal with the noxious stimulus. In the case of anger, he is more concerned with the violation of rights, rules, and principles and with the blameworthiness of the offensive agent, and less so with the danger to himself.

The typical ideation leading to either anxiety, sadness, euphoria or anger has a counterpart in the characteristic ideation found in anxiety reactions, depression, mania, and paranoid states, respectively. A significant difference between psychological disorders and normal emotional responses is that the ideational content of the disorders contains a consistent distortion of a realistic situation. Whereas the normal emotional response is based on a reasonable appraisal of the reality situation, the responses in psychological disturbances are determined to a far greater degree by internal (that is, psychological) factors that confound the appraisal of reality.

CHAPTER 4

Cognitive Content of the Emotional Disorders

The neurotic is not only emotionally sick—he is cognitively wrong. —Abraham Maslow

The capacity of human beings to integrate myriad environmental events and to react adaptively is a tribute to our psychological development. Even more striking is our ability to discriminate among the subtle cues in interpersonal situations and our resiliency in the face of disappointment and frustration. The ability to use imagination creatively and yet to check it from impinging on our sense of reality is further evidence of our maturation.

Despite this glowing picture, it is obvious that we do not respond consistently well to all challenges. We have specific vulnerabilities, "fault lines" along which stresses accumulate and may set off tremors or eruptions—behavior commonly labeled "over-reacting." Under such conditions unrealistic appraisals override realistic appraisals, and we may realize that our reactions are largely irrational.

We are all familiar with examples of over-reacting:

A man suddenly becomes belligerent when his friends question his role as an authority in a particular area; a generally self-composed woman becomes very upset when she finds "she doesn't have a thing to wear" to a formal dinner; a student who receives a lower grade than expected on an examination becomes morose and considers himself a total failure. Such instances of excessive or inappropriate emotional reactions point to the importance of the internal dramas that permeate our experiences: We envision clashes of the forces of good and evil, triumphs and tragedies, heroics and infamies. We have glimpses of these internal theatricals in our dreams and daydreams. When the dramatic force of these productions sweeps over our rational appraisals, we experience excessive or inappropriate emotional reactions.

Some people become so engulfed by these internally generated fantasies that their behavior and emotions are controlled by the fantasies. When the inappropriate or excessive reactions burgeon beyond a certain point or level of distress or disability, then we are likely to label them "emotional disorder," "neurosis," "psychological disturbance," or "psychiatric disease." These disorders frequently assume a characteristic form that allows them to be fitted into a generally recognized category such as depression, anxiety state, or paranoid state. Although related to the kinds of emotional reactions already described (Chapter 3), these psychological disorders differ from normal emotional reactions because of the intrusion of unrealistic thinking regarding key issues in the patient's life. The disturbance in thinking can be best illustrated by one of the most dramatic syndromes seen by therapists—acute neurosis.

THE ACUTE EMOTIONAL DISTURBANCE

The misery of psychiatric disorders is epitomized by the acute neurotic reaction. In its most flagrant form, this reaction is manifested by a variety of intense, unpleasant experiences. Familiar objects seem strange, distorted, or unreal. Moreover, the patient's internal experiences seem peculiar. He may experience loss of normal sensation in his limbs or in the interior of his body. His body may feel heavy or weightless. Events take on new meanings and significances. A past occurrence previously regarded as trivial looms large. Such reactions are generally beyond the realm of the patient's ordinary experience. Some patients compare the strangeness of the experience to reactions while undergoing anesthesia, having a "bad trip" under the influence of drugs, or having a nightmare.

A devastating aspect of the acute emotional disturbance is the slippage of controls previously taken for granted. The patient has to grapple to retain voluntary control over concentration, attention, and focusing. He has trouble framing his thoughts or following along a consistent line of thinking. His awareness of himself and of his surroundings is not only altered, but diminished, so that he has difficulty in perceiving many details in his environment. Paradoxically, however, he may be exquisitely sensitive to such stimuli as the tone of a person's voice or certain internal sensations. He may be confused to the point of disorientation. Even though he may correctly identify who he is and where he is, he is not positive of this identification.

The extreme form of this disturbance has been labeled a "catastrophic reaction." The person expresses his uncanny experiences by descriptions such as, "I don't feel that I'm really here," "I feel different," "Things look different." In trying to capture the quality of the experience, he applies terms such as, "I feel I am losing my grip;" "I am going out of my mind;" "I am dying;" "I feel I am ready to pass out;" "I am coming apart;" "I am going crazy." Although these eerie feelings are often interpreted by the afflicted as a sign that he is "going insane," they are generally associated with acute neurotic reactions rather than with psychosis.

In addition to experiencing the strange feelings and disruption of ordinary psychological processes described above, the patient may be engulfed by intense anxiety, sadness, or rage. Even when the emotion is a magnification of a pleasant feeling, such as the euphoria of manic reactions, its intensity makes it unpleasant.

Is it possible to make sense out of the strange psychological phenomena in an acute neurosis? A striking component of the peculiar experiences is intense self-consciousness. The patient becomes overly aware of his internal processes. His attention is fixed on his perceptions, thoughts, and feelings, with the result that these psychological processes become extremely vivid. In addition, he is overly attentive to certain cues in his environment and oblivious to others—"tunnel vision." With the binding of his attention to specific internal and external stimuli, the patient has great difficulty in mobilizing sufficient attention to focus on other areas of experience.

The phenomenon of self-consciousness and attention-binding in acute neurosis is similar to reactions experienced by many people in realistically threatening situations. A student taking an important oral or written examination may experience anxiety because of the threat to his life objectives. He finds it difficult to focus on his immediate task—reading or listening to the questions and drawing on his memory to supply the answers. His attention is drawn, instead, to ideas about failing, continual evaluations of his performance, and scanning of his unpleasant emotional state. Because of the fixation of his attention on these distracting ideas, he has difficulty in making sense out of the questions, and he experiences "blocking" in his attempts to recall material and to form the appropriate sentences. His blocking and impaired efficiency are produced not by the anxiety per se, but by the binding of his attention to irrelevant thoughts and feelings.[1]

A similar set of psychological reactions may ensue upon exposure to physical danger. A soldier exposed to combat for the first time may experience difficulties in concentration and in shifting his focus. His attention may be so fixed on the notion of danger and the wish to escape that he is unable to understand and follow commands that will protect his life. Similar experiences are reported by people in other precarious situations. A novice, hiking along a steep mountain slope, may be so preoccupied with the notion of falling that he walks clumsily or stumbles, thus placing himself in jeopardy.

Compare the reactions to realistic threats with those experienced by a patient with an acute anxiety neurosis. The patient, similarly, is overly alert to stimuli relevant to danger; any change in his environment, such as an unexpected sound, draws his attention: He is overly vigilant to any signal that might be indicative of danger. At the same time, he has difficulty in focusing his attention on

[1]For experimental validation, see Sarason (1972b) and Horowitz et al. (1971).

those components of his environment that do not denote danger.

Despite the similarities, the patient with acute anxiety reaction differs significantly from the person exposed to a realistic threat. The danger the patient perceives is nonexistent or blown out of proportion. He is not only preoccupied with the idea of danger, but he consistently misinterprets innocuous stimuli as indicative of danger.

The problem of the anxiety-neurotic is not primarily in labeling stimuli—he can readily label a loud sound—but in the meanings and significances he attaches to certain stimuli. His interpretations tend to be far-fetched, improbable, unrealistic. The sound of a siren indicates his house is on fire; a pain in the back of his head suggests he is having a stroke; an approaching stranger is regarded as an assailant. The cumulative effect of indiscriminately interpreting events as danger signals is a warped view of the real world and escalating anxiety. The misconstruing of situations constitutes cognitive distortion ranging from mild inaccuracy to gross misinterpretation.

Binding of attention, constriction of awareness, selective abstraction, and distortion occur not only in acute anxiety neuroses but in other acute neuroses such as depression, hypomania, and paranoid state. These states differ in the kind of emotion experienced: sadness, euphoria, anger. The differences in the emotion may be accounted for by the differences in the deviant meanings or the themes of the thinking. As we shall see, in each neurosis reality is twisted to fit concepts that dominate the patient's thinking. Thinking disorders are also at the core of other neuroses such as hysteria, phobia, and obsessive-compulsive neurosis.

NEUROTIC DISORDERS

Although the acute emotional disturbance is not observed frequently by clinicians, its florid characteristics illuminate the more subtle difficulties encountered in the more common forms of neurotic reaction. In the less dramatic forms of neurosis, the thinking disturbance may occur only in certain situations or in relation to specific problems that impinge on the patient's vulnerabilities. In other situations, his thinking is reasonably attuned to reality. Nonetheless, even the more chronic or milder forms of the neuroses are occasionally punctuated by episodes similar to the acute emotional disturbance.

Since canalized thinking, attention-fixation, and distortions of reality may occur in all the neuroses, the key differences among the neuroses are revealed in the *content* of the aberrant thinking rather than in its form. Later we shall review other thinking peculiarities typical of the neuroses in general, but for the present we shall examine the differences in the content.

In those neuroses characterized by excessive emotional reactions, the emotional state characteristic of each disorder is evoked by the specific content of the aberrant thinking. Sadness—the typical emotion of depression—stems from the patient's tendency to interpret his experiences in terms of being deprived, deficient, or defeated. The euphoria observed in hypomanic states results from the perseverative preoccupation with ideas of self-enhancement. The anxious patient experiences his feelings of distress by overinterpreting his experiences in terms of danger, while the paranoid patient feels intense anger because of his fixation on notions of being abused.

The basic data for ascertaining the thinking disorder

in neurotic patients were derived from verbatim notes of their verbal reports during psychotherapy or formal psychoanalysis (Beck 1963; 1967). These reports dealt with their major repetitive ideas, their descriptions of their interpretations of situations, and their automatic thoughts. The possibility that I may have influenced the nature of the patients' reports is minimized by the fact that my own preconceptions were contrary to the content that emerged. For instance, the repeated observation that depressed feelings and anxiety were based on cognitive distortions relevant to the theme of loss or danger, respectively, forced me to revise my thinking about these conditions. The new formulations gradually eased out the psychoanalytic theories that I had been taught and believed: that depression is caused by hostility turned against the self and anxiety is stimulated by the threatened break into consciousness of a taboo wish.

I initially reported my findings and conclusions based on 81 patients treated by me (Beck, 1963). The findings held for a later sample of 100 patients in treatment with me (Beck, 1970c). I also found that, by asking relevant questions during diagnostic interviews of patients in the clinic, the psychiatric residents obtained further confirmatory material. Concomitantly, I found support for the formulations in a number of controlled investigations by my research group (Beck, 1961; Loeb, Beck, and Diggory, 1971) and in independent observations and studies by other clinicians and researchers (Ellis, 1962; Velten, 1967).

On the basis of the clinical observations and systematic studies, I was able to distinguish among the common neurotic disorders according to differences in the content of ideation. These differences are illustrated in the following table.

TABLE 1

IDEATIONAL CONTENT OF NEUROTIC DISORDERS

	Idiosyncratic Ideational Content
Depression	Devaluation of domain
Hypomania	Inflated evaluation of domain
Anxiety Neurosis	Danger to domain
Phobia	Danger connected with specific, avoidable situations
Paranoid State	Unjustified intrusion on domain
Hysteria	Concept of motor or sensory abnormality
Obsession	Warning or doubting
Compulsion	Self-command to perform specific act to ward off danger

DEPRESSION

The thought content of depressed patients centers on a significant loss. The patient perceives that he has lost something he considers essential to his happiness or tranquility; he anticipates negative outcomes from any important undertaking; and he regards himself as deficient in the attributes necessary for achieving important goals. This theme may be formulated in terms of the cognitive triad: a negative conception of the self, a negative interpretation of life experiences, and a nihilistic view of the future.

The sense of irreversible loss and negative expectation leads to the typical emotions associated with depression: sadness, disappointment, and apathy. Furthermore, as the sense of being trapped in an unpleasant situtation or of being enmeshed in insoluble problems increases, spontaneous constructive motivation dissipates. The patient, moreover, feels impelled to escape from the apparently intolerable condition via suicide.

HYPOMANIC STATE

The thought content of the hypomanic or manic patient is the reverse of that of the depressive. The manic or hypomanic patient perceives a significant gain in each of his life experiences. He indiscriminately attributes positive values to his experiences, unrealistically expects favorable results from his endeavors, and has exaggerated ideas of his abilities. These positive evaluations lead to feelings of euphoria. Moreover, the continued bombardment of inflated self-evaluations and overly optimistic expectations energizes and propels him into continuous activity.

ANXIETY NEUROSIS

The thinking of the anxious patient is dominated by themes of danger to his domain; that is, he anticipates detrimental occurences to himself, his family, his property, or to his status and to other intangibles he values. In contrast to the phobic patient who experiences anxiety in avoidable situations, the anxiety-neurotic perceives danger in situations he cannot avoid. A person who is continuously afraid of developing a serious or fatal illness may interpret any unusual physiological symptom as a sign of such illness. Shortness of breath may arouse the idea that he is having a heart attack; diarrhea, constipation, or a vague pain may lead him to believe he has cancer. Frequently, his fears envelop external stimuli. He may interpret any unexpected sound as a signal of disaster. Noises in his house arouse fears of burglars breaking in; automobile backfire suggests gunshots; a youngster's shout stimulates visions of physical violence.

Many anxious patients are afraid predominantly of

psychological harm. The anxious person is often concerned that other people, strangers as well as friends, will reject, humiliate, or depreciate him. Anticipation of physical or psychological harm is chained to anxiety; consequently, when such expectations are formed, anxiety is stimulated.

PHOBIA

In phobias, the anticipation of physical or psychological harm is confined to definable situations. If the patient can avoid these situations, then he does not feel threatened and may be tranquil. If he enters into these situations because of necessity or because of his own desire to overcome his problem, he experiences the typical subjective and physiological symptoms of the anxiety-neurotic.

As in the psychiatric disturbances described previously, the patient's cognitive response to the stimulus situation may be expressed in purely verbal form or in the form of imagery. A woman with a fear of heights, who ventured to the twentieth floor of a building, promptly had a visual image of the floor tilting, of sliding toward the window, and of falling out. She experienced intense anxiety, as though the image were an actual external event.

Fears of particular situations are based on the patient's exaggerated conception of specific harmful attributes of these situations. A person with a tunnel phobia will experience fears that the tunnel will collapse on him, that he will suffocate, or that he will have an acute, life-threatening illness and be unable to get help in time to save him. The acrophobic similarly reacts to high places with fears that he might fall off, that the structure will collapse, or that he might jump off impulsively.

PARANOID STATE

The paranoid patient perseverates in assuming that other people are deliberately abusing him or interfering with his objectives. Unlike the depressed patient who feels that supposed insults or rejections are justified, the paranoid patient is preoccupied with the idea that an injustice has been done. The main theme in his thinking is "I am right, he is wrong," in contrast to the depressed patient who follows the theme, "I am wrong, he is right." Unlike depressed patients, the paranoid patient does not experience any lowering of his self-esteem. He is more concerned with the injustice of the attack on his domain than with the actual loss to his domain.

Differences among anxiety neurosis, neurotic depression, and paranoid state may be summarized as follows: The anxious patient focuses on the possibility of an attack; the paranoid patient concentrates on the injustice or malevolent motives behind a supposed attack or infringement on his boundaries; the depressed patient focuses on the presumed loss he attributes to some inadequacy of his own.

OBSESSIONS AND COMPULSIONS

The content of obsessions is generally concerned with some remote risk or danger expressed in the form of a doubt or warning. The person may continually doubt whether he has performed an act necessary to ensure his safety (for example, turning off a gas oven), or he may doubt whether he will be able to perform adequately. The thoughts differ from those of the anxiety-neurotic in that they are concerned with an action the patient believes he should have taken or an action he should not have taken. As an example of the latter, a patient repeatedly had the thought that he might have contracted leukemia because he touched the garment of a leukemic victim.

Compulsions consist of attempts to allay excessive doubts or obsessions through action. A hand-washing compulsion, for instance, is based on the patient's notion that he has not removed all the dirt or contaminants from parts of his body. He regards the dirt as a source of danger, either as a cause of physical disease or as a source of offensive odors. We often see the triad of phobia-obsession-compulsion. A patient, for example, was afraid of being harmed by radiation. His phobia was manifested by avoiding contact with objects that might emit radiation (e.g., clocks, because of radioactive dials; or television sets). After an unavoidable contact with such an object, he ruminated about the possibility of contamination (obsession). This led him to taking frequent, prolonged baths to remove the presumed radioactive material (compulsion).

HYSTERICAL REACTIONS

In hysteria the patient believes he has a physical disorder. Since the imagined disorder is not fatal, he tends to accept it without severe anxiety. Patients with hysteria are essentially "sensory imagers"; that is, they imagine the particular illness and then take the sensory experience as corroborative evidence of having the illness. The patient typically experiences sensory or motor abnormalities that fit the pattern of his erroneous concept of organic pathology.

PSYCHOSES

Although the complicated subject of psychoses is beyond the scope of our inquiry, it might be useful to compare the thought content of psychoses with that of neuroses. The ideational themes of psychotic depression are analogous to those of neurotic depression. Paranoia or paranoid schizophrenia shows a similar content to that of paranoid states. The manic reaction resembles the broad content of the hypomanic. The content of the ideation of the psychoses, however, is more bizarre, grotesque, and extreme than that of the neuroses. Whereas a neurotic depressive may view himself as being socially inadequate, the psychotic depressive may believe he emits disgusting odors that alienate other people.

Psychoses as a class show more pronounced cognitive impairment than do neuroses. The perseverative ideation is more intense and less subject to modification through corrective experience. The patient's capacity to view his erroneous ideas objectively is much more limited; furthermore, the degree of illogical and unrealistic thinking is more pronounced.

NATURE OF THINKING DISORDERS

A thinking disorder, in the absence of organic pathology, has generally been considered a feature of schizophrenia. In contrast, depression, mania, and anxiety—with their florid emotional manifestations—have been regarded, in essence, as "affective" or emotional disorders. However, there is now considerable evidence that a disorder in thinking, less gross and more circumscribed than that described in schizophrenia, is an important component of the common psychiatric syndromes.

In a long-term study (Beck, 1963) I found that each of the patients systematically misconstrued specific kinds of experiences. These distortions of reality ranged from subtle inaccuracies in the mild neurotics to the familiar grotesque misinterpretations and delusions in the psychotics. The peculiar ideation of the patients showed systematic departures from reality and logic, including arbitrary inferences, selective abstractions, and overgeneralizations. These distortions occurred in ideation that was relevant to the patient's specific problem. For example, the depressed patient showed aberrations when he was thinking about his worth; the anxious patient, when he was concerned with the notion of danger.

The distorted ideas had the characteristics of "automatic thoughts" (see Chapter 2). They appeared to arise as if by reflex, without any apparent antecedent reflection or reasoning. They seemed plausible to the patient even though implausible to other people. Finally, they were less amenable to change by reason or contradictory evidence than were other forms of ideation not associated with the specific form of psychopathology. I observed a gradation of impaired thinking from the mild neurotic to severe psychotic. As the illness became intensified, the patient showed a progressively greater degree of distortion, increasing repetition of distorted ideas, and progressive fixation of the distortions.

PERSONALIZATION

The inevitable egocentricity of man has intrigued writers and philosophers for ages. In a sense, everybody seems to have a private world of which he is the axis. Heidegger (1927) and other have described how each individual constructs his own personal world. Nonetheless, people are generally capable of making objective judgments about external events—or even about themselves—and are able to disentangle the personal meaning of an event from its objective characteristics. They are able to make judgments on two different levels—one relevant to themselves (or their domain), and the other detached from themselves. In psychiatric disorders, we find that the egocentric interpretations become unusually compelling and may totally displace objective judgments. Labels such as "personalization" or "self-reference" are applied to the propensity to interpret events in terms of their personal meanings.

The process of personalization or self-reference can be best illustrated by a few extreme examples: specifically, patients who fall into the loose category of "psychotic." A paranoid schizophrenic patient believed that the images he saw on the television screen were talking directly to him, and he spoke back to them. A psychotic depressive heard about an epidemic of an infectious disease in a distant land and blamed himself for having caused it. A manic woman believed that everybody she passed on the street was in love with her. Psychotic patients consistently interpret events totally unrelated to them as though they were caused by them or directed against them.

Less extreme forms of self-reference are found in neurotic patients. They tend to overestimate the degree to which events are related to them and to be excessively absorbed in the personal meanings of particular happenings. A depressed patient, observing a frown on another person's face, thinks, "He is disgusted with me." Although it is conceivable that in this instance the patient's judgment is correct, his error lies in his notion that every grimace he observes in other people represents disgust with him. He overinterprets the frequency as well as the degree of negative feelings he evokes in other people. A depressed mother blames herself for every imperfection in her children. An anxious patient relates every danger signal to himself: A passing ambulance makes him think his child has had an accident.

Another form of personalization is found in man's irrepressible tendency to compare himself with other people. A woman observing a billboard of a happy mother and child thinks, "She's a much more devoted mother than I." A student, hearing that another student has won a prize, thinks, "I must be dumb or I would have won the prize." A young phobic patient, reading of an elderly person having a heart attack, thinks, "If he had a heart attack, it could happen to *me*" and starts to feel pain in his chest.

The basic egocentric coloring may be found in each of the facets of aberrant thinking of neurotic patients. The process of decentering, that is, training the individual to use a frame of reference that does not pivot on him, is described in Chapter 10.

POLARIZED THINKING

The neurotic patient is prone to think in extremes in situations that impinge on his sensitive areas, for example, his self-evaluations (depression), the possibility of personal danger (anxiety neurosis). Thinking in extremes may be confined to only a few areas. Events are labeled as black or white, good or bad, wonderful or horrible. This characteristic has been termed "dichotomous thinking" or "bipolar thinking" (Neuringer, 1961). The basic premises underlying this kind of thinking are generally couched in absolute terms such as "always" or "never."

An example from everyday life is a young man who was fixated on the concept of absolute acceptance and rejection. He would scrutinize practically everybody with whom he came in contact—a clerk in a department store, a passerby in the street—to determine whether the person appeared to accept or reject him. He could not modulate his judgment to include fine gradations such as mild acceptance, mild rejection, or neutrality. Neutrality (and indifference) represented rejection and made him feel sad; a smile represented complete acceptance and elicited euphoria.

A similar example of this kind of thinking was exhibited by a young college student when he played basketball. If he scored less than eight points in a game, he thought, "I'm a failure," and he felt sad. Scoring eight points or more meant, "I'm really a great player," and led to feelings of exhilaration.

Sometimes thinking in extremes is unipolar: for example, events may be perceived either as totally bad or neutral or irrelevant. "Catastrophizing," a common characteristic of anxious patients, illustrates anticipation of extreme adverse outcomes. The thinking of the anxious patient is grooved toward considering the most unfavorable of all possible outcomes of a situation. For example, a patient who received a scratch on his arm immediately began to dwell on the possibility of its leading to a fatal infection.

One's penchant to make extreme judgments may be confined to tangible objects. A man, for example, became upset when he detected the slightest damage in his material possessions. A slight dent in his car, a scratch on his furniture, a worn spot on his clothes represented major losses. On one occasion, he discovered that an unexpectedly large flame in his fireplace had scorched the protective grille. He was agitated for several hours. His thoughts were: "This is a permanent defacement, it can't be repaired. It ruins the whole room, it was perfect before, now it's wrecked." As the days passed, he viewed the damage more objectively (that is, as trivial). Also the degree to which he exaggerated the damage was reflected in his self-criticisms, "I was a fool to let it happen, I am inept, I never do anything right."

Persons who characteristically react to a noxious stimulus with anger may also show extreme judgments. Consider this reaction of a parent whose child had lost a glove: "That's terrible. You'll drive us to the poorhouse. You never do anything right."

Related to making extreme global judgments are other types of thinking that lead to distortions or misinterpretations (Beck, 1963). *Selective abstraction* refers to abstracting a detail out of context, and thus, missing the significance of the total situation. A person makes an *arbitrary inference* when he jumps to a conclusion when evidence is lacking or is actually contrary to the conclusion. *Overgeneralization* refers to unjustified generalization on the basis of a single incident. For example, a child makes a single mistake and thinks, "I never do anything right." These examples illustrate how aberrant thinking is aroused in situations that impinge on specific vulnerabilities, such as acceptance-rejection, success-failure, health-sickness, or gain-loss.

"THE LAW OF RULES"

We have seen (in Chapter 2) that a person has a program of rules according to which he deciphers and evaluates his experiences and regulates his behavior and that of others. These rules operate without the person's being aware of his rule-book. He screens selectively, integrates, and sorts the flow of stimuli and forms his own responses without articulating to himself the rules and concepts that dictate his interpretations and reactions. The operation of the input-output apparatus is far from perfect.

Problems inevitably crop up in understanding the behavior of other people. Because of his having been inadequately or inappropriately prepared by his previous experience, a person may infer incorrect *meanings* from their behavior: their underlying attitudes towards him, their present intentions, their probable future conduct toward him.

In a previous example (Chapter 2), a student is corrected by an instructor. The student wonders: Is this a friendly gesture? Or does it mean that he has irritated the instructor? Does it indicate that the instructor believes that the student is stupid? Is the instructor likely to be harsh and punitive in grading him? With this wide range of possible inferences from a particular interaction, it is not surprising that many students are hypersensitive to teachers' comments!

At times a student may read more harshness into a teacher's comment than was intended. If the student's exaggerations or distortions of the interaction are mild and transient, then he can maintain his psychological equilibrium. However, let us consider a bright student who, because of his particular sensitivities, is predisposed to regard criticisms as derogatory. As "criticisms" accumulate, he becomes increasingly more likely to label subsequent remarks or suggestions by the teacher in the same way. Unless his tendency is reversed by some clearly positive action by the teacher, he becomes overly inclusive in his labeling: He begins to regard neutral or mildly positive messages from the teacher as derogatory. He overgeneralizes so that he concludes that not only this teacher, but all his teachers, are critical and believe he is stupid. He proceeds on the basis of this "evidence" to the conclusion that he is totally, irreversibly defective—worthless. Further, picture the student back in his room ruminating about these "denunciations" and "errors" to the point that he is no longer able to concentrate on his work. He then interprets his difficulties in concentrating and subsequent impaired performance in his classwork as evidence of his defectiveness. Now include the inevitable dysphoria—probably sadness mixed with anxiety—and we have the beginnings of a psychiatric disorder. If the condition persists for many days or weeks, it becomes depression.

We can analyze this hypothetical case in terms of the student's rule book. In every classroom interaction, the student repetitively applies rules regarding the teacher's evaluations. He uses the following rules: "A criticism means the teacher thinks I'm stupid. If an authority thinks that I'm stupid, it means I *am* stupid. Since I am stupid, I shall never get anywhere." He then applies a formula to his impaired performance: "My inefficiency *proves* I'm stupid." He even has a rule for the consequent dysphoria: "If I'm sad it means that things won't work out for me." The student is applying a series of "logical" operations with the conclusion of one constituting a premise for the next conclusion.

Each of the psychiatric disorders previously discussed has its own set of rules. In anxiety neurosis, the rules are concerned with the concept of danger and the patient's estimate of his capacity for coping with it. The conclusions derived from the application of the rules take the form of predictions such as, "I am in imminent danger of losing my most prized attributes (health, life, friend, job)." "I do not have the means to ward off this danger." The specific rules leading to these conclusions are applied (or misapplied) to specific events: "My rapid heartbeat means I'm having a heart attack, and I may die if I don't get help." "If I am away from home, calamities may occur and I won't be able to cope with them." "If I make a mistake, I may antagonize my boss and he will fire me."

In anxiety, the rules are generally conditional: "*If* a particular event occurs, it will probably have adverse results." Hence, when the event occurs, there is still a possibility of an innocuous outcome. In contrast, the rules in depression are absolute and unconditional: "My present deficiencies mean I shall always be a failure."

In phobias, the rules are also conditional; they apply to situations the patient is successfully able to avoid: "If I go into a tunnel, I might suffocate." "If I go to an unfamiliar place, I might get lost." In these cases, the patient also operates under the rule, "I won't be able to cope with the situation myself." As in the case of anxiety, these rules attach a high probability of disaster occurring. However, the patient is often fortified by the assumption, "If a helpful person is with me, he can save me." Hence, many phobic patients can enter the frightening situation if a "helper" is available.

In depression, the rules as formulated derive negative meanings and negative predictions from a present or past circumstance. There is no "escape clause" as in anxiety and phobias. Examples of the rules are: "Not being successful in my career equals being a total failure." "Since I am sad now, I shall always be sad." "When something goes wrong, it is my fault." "Losing my wife's love means I am worthless." "Not being admired means I am unlikable."

In manic conditions, the content of the assumptions is opposite to that in depression. The rules are framed in such a way as to exaggerate the gain and elevate self-esteem: "When people look at me, they admire me." "If I have a job to do, I shall do a superb job." "Each success proves again how superior I am."

The rules of the paranoid patient are likely to be unconditional and absolute. The content of the rules reeks of conspiracies, unjustified abuse, discrimination: "When people don't agree with me, they are deliberately trying to oppose me." "When I don't get what I want, it means somebody has sabotaged me." "When things don't go right, it is because of other people's interference."

When we question a patient about his ideas, he generally does not volunteer the rule that shapes his interpretation of events. Instead, he states his *conclusion*. For example, a patient with anxiety neurosis states, "I may be about to die"; with depression, "I have lost everything that matters to me . . . I am worthless"; with mania, "I am supreme"; with paranoid reaction, "Everyone is against me."

We have to work back from the conclusion to derive the rule (assumption, premise). Sometimes, the patient is able to articulate the rule without difficulty. A depressed, suicidal woman who had previously had a breech in her relationship with her lover said, "I am worthless." When asked why, she stated, as though it were a universal truth, "If I don't have love, I am worthless." More frequently, a sequence of questions is necessary to elicit the rule:

> *Anxious patient:* "I think I am dying."
> *Therapist:* "What makes you think so?"
> *Patient:* "My heart is beating hard. Things seem blurred. I can't catch my breath . . . I am sweating all over."
> *Therapist:* "Why does that mean you are dying?"
> *Patient:* "Because this is what it is like to die."
> *Therapist:* "How do you know?"
> *Patient:* [after some reflection] "I guess I don't know. But I *think* these are signs of dying."

The patient's rule (premise) is that this combination of symptoms equals imminent death. In actuality, however, the signs (palpitations, difficulty in focusing, shortness of breath) are typical signs of an acute anxiety attack. (It is true, of course, that if associated with typical signs of organic disease the "anxiety symptoms" might be indicators of a serious threat to life.) The patient's ideation and anxiety become involved in a vicious cycle. Thoughts of dying lead to increasing anxiety, as manifested by the physiological symptoms; these symptoms, in turn, are interpreted as signs of imminent death.

How do these rules hypertrophy into an emotional

disturbance? Since the rules tend to be couched in extreme words, they lead to an extreme conclusion. They are applied as though in a syllogism.

Major premise: "If I don't have love, I am worthless."
Special case: "Raymond doesn't love me."
Conclusion: "I am worthless."

Of course, the patient does not report a sequence of thoughts in the form of a syllogism. The major premise (rule) is already part of his cognitive organization and is applied to the presenting circumstances. The patient may ruminate over the minor premise (the specific situation) and is certainly conscious of the conclusion.

The thinking disorder characteristic of psychological disturbance may be analyzed in terms of the operation of the rules. Such characteristic thinking aberrations as exaggeration, overgeneralization, and absoluteness are built into the framework of the rule and, consequently, press the person to make an exaggerated, overgeneralized, absolute conclusion. (Of course, in normal states, there are also more flexible rules, which tend to mitigate the more extreme rules that are prepotent in states of disturbance.) When the theme of the patient's preoccupation is related to his specific sensitivities, the more primitive rules tend to displace the more mature concepts. Once the patient accepts the validity of an extreme conclusion, he is more susceptible to an ever-increasing expansion of the primitive rules.

If, for instance, he succumbs to the notion, "Since my friends did not call me today, they regard me as unlovable and worthless," he may be drawn to accept this conclusion as the premise for a more far-reaching one: "Since I am worthless, nobody will ever like me." This premise sets the stage for the following conclusion: "Without love, life is not worth living. Therefore, there is no point to my continuing to live."

CHAPTER 5

The Paradoxes of Depression

Lying awake, calculating the future,
Trying to unweave, unwind, unravel
And piece together the past and the future,
Between midnight and dawn, when the past is
all deception,
The future futureless. . . . —T. S. Eliot

A scientist, shortly after assuming the presidency of a prestigious scientific group, gradually became morose and confided to a friend that he had an overwhelming urge to leave his career and become a hobo.

A devoted mother who had always felt strong love for her children started to neglect them and formulated a serious plan to destroy them and then herself.

An epicurean who relished eating beyond all other satisfactions developed an aversion to food and stopped eating.

A woman, upon hearing of the sudden death of a close friend, emitted the first smile in several weeks.

These strange actions, completely inconsistent with the individual's previous behavior and values, are all expressions of the same underlying condition—depression. By what perversity does depression mock the most hallowed notions of human nature and biology?

The instinct for self-preservation and the maternal instincts appear to vanish. Basic biological drives such as hunger and sexual urge are extinguished. Sleep, the easer of all woes, is thwarted. "Social instincts," such as attraction to other people, love, and affection evaporate. The pleasure principle and reality principle, the goals of maximizing pleasure and minimizing pain, are turned around. Not only is the capacity for enjoyment stifled, but the victims of this odd malady appear driven to behave in ways that enhance their suffering. The depressed person's capacity to respond with mirth to humorous situations or with anger to situations that would ordinarily infuriate him seems lost.

At one time, this strange affliction was ascribed to demons that allegedly took possession of the victim. Theories advanced since that time have not yet provided a durable solution to the problem of depression. We are still encumbered by a psychological disorder that seems to discredit the most firmly entrenched concepts of the nature of man. Paradoxically, the anomalies of depression may provide clues for understanding this mysterious condition.

The complete reversal in the depressed patient's behavior seems, initially, to defy explanation. During his depression, the patient's manifest personality is far more like that of other depressives than his own previous personality. Feelings of pleasure and joy are replaced by sadness and apathy; the broad range of spontaneous desires and involvement in activities are eclipsed by passivity and desires to escape; hunger and sexual drive are replaced by revulsion toward food and sex; interest and involvement in usual activities are converted into avoidance and withdrawal. Finally, the desire to live is switched off and replaced by the wish to die.

As an initial step in understanding depression, we can attempt to arrange the various phenomena into some kind of understandable sequence. Various writers have assigned primacy to one of the following: intense sadness, wishes to "hibernate," self-destructive wishes, or physiological disturbance.

Is the painful emotion the catalytic agent? If depression is a primary affective disorder, it should be possible to account for the other symptoms on the basis of the emotional state. However, the unpleasant subjective state in itself does not appear to be an adequate stimulus for the other depressive symptoms. Other states of suffering such as physical pain, nausea, dizziness, shortness of breath, or anxiety rarely lead to symptoms typical of depression such as renunciation of major objectives in life, obliteration of affectionate feelings, or the wish to die. On the contrary, people suffering physical pain seem to treasure more than ever those aspects of life they have found meaningful. Moreover, the state of sadness does not have qualities we would expect to produce the self-castigations, distortions in thinking, and loss of drive for gratifications characteristic of depression.

Similar problems are raised in assigning primacy to other aspects of depression. Some writers have latched onto the passivity and withdrawal of attachments to other people to advance the notion that depression results from an atavistic wish to hibernate. If the goal of depression is to conserve energy, however, why is the patient driven to castigate himself and engage in continuous, aimless activities when agitated? Why does he seek to destroy himself—the source of energy?

Ascribing the primary role to the physiological symptoms such as disturbances in sleep, appetite, and sexuality also poses problems. It is difficult to understand the sequence by which these physiological disturbances lead to such varied phenomena as self-criticisms, the negative view of the world, and loss of the anger and mirth responses. Certainly, physiological responses such as loss of appetite and sleep resulting from an acute physical illness do not lead to other components of the depressive constellation.

THE CLUE: THE SENSE OF LOSS

The task of sorting the phenomena of depression into an understandable sequence may be simplified by asking the patient what he feels sad about and by encouraging him to express his repetitive ideas. Depressed patients generally provide essential information in spontaneous statements such as: "I'm sad because I'm worthless"; "I have no future"; "I've lost everything"; "My family is gone"; "I have nobody"; "Life has nothing for me." It is relatively easy to detect the dominant theme in the statements of the moderately or severely depressed patient. *He regards himself as lacking some element or attribute that he considers essential for his happiness:* competence in attaining his goals, attractiveness to other people, closeness to family or friends, tangible possessions, good health, status or position. Such self-appraisals reflect the way the depressed patient perceives his life situation.

In exploring the theme of loss, we find that the psychological disorder revolves around a cognitive problem. The depressed patient shows specific distortions. He has a negative view of his world, a negative concept of himself, and a negative appraisal of his future: the *cognitive triad.*

The distorted evaluations concern shrinkage of his domain, and lead to sadness (Chapter 3). The depressive's conception of his valued attributes, relationships, and achievements is saturated with the notion of loss—past, present, and future. When he considers his present position, he sees a barren world; he feels pressed to the wall by external demands that cheat him of his meager resources and keep him from attaining what he wants.

The term "loser" captures the flavor of the depressive's appraisal of himself and his experience. He agonizes over the notion that he has experienced significant losses, such as his friends, his health, his prized possessions. He also regards himself as a "loser" in the colloquial sense: He is a misfit—an inferior and an inadequate being who is unable to meet his responsibilities and attain his goals. If he undertakes a project or seeks some gratification, he expects to be defeated or disappointed. He finds no respite during sleep. He has repetitive dreams in which he is a misfit, a failure.

In considering the concept of loss, we should be sensitive to the crucial importance of meanings and connotations. What represents a painful loss for one person may be regarded as trivial by another. It is important to recognize that the depressed patient dwells on hypothetical losses and pseudo losses. When he thinks about a potential loss, he regards the possibility as though it were an accomplished fact. A depressed man, for example, characteristically reacted to his wife's tardiness in meeting him with the thought, "She might have died on the way." He then construed the hypothetical loss as an actual event and became forlorn. Pseudo loss refers to the incorrect labeling of any event as a loss; for example, a change in status that may in actuality be a gain. A depressed patient who sold some shares of stock at a large profit experienced a prolonged sense of deprivation over eliminating the securities from his portfolio; he ruminated over the notion that the sale had impoverished him.

Granted that the perception of loss produces feelings of sadness, how does this sense of loss engender other symptoms of depression: pessimism, self-criticism, escape-avoidance-giving up, suicidal wishes, and physiological disorders?

In order to answer this question, it would be useful to explore the chronology of depression, the onset and full development of symptoms. This sequence is most clearly demonstrated in cases of "reactive depression," that is, depression in which there is a clear-cut precipitating factor. Other cases of depression, in which the onset is more insidious, show similar (although more subtle) patterns.

DEVELOPMENT OF DEPRESSION

In the course of his development, the depression-prone person may become sensitized by certain unfavorable types of life situations, such as the loss of a parent or chronic rejection by his peers. Other unfavorable conditions of a less obvious nature may similarly produce vulnerability to depression. These traumatic experiences predispose the person to overreact to analogous conditions later in life. He has a tendency to make extreme, absolute judgments when such situations occur. A loss is viewed as irrevocable; indifference, as total rejection.

Other depression-prone people set rigid, perfectionistic goals for themselves during childhood, so that their universe collapses when they confront inevitable disappointments later in life.[1]

The stresses responsible for adult depressions impinge on the person's specific vulnerability. Numerous clinical and research reports agree on the following types of precipitating events: the disruption of a relationship with a person to whom the patient is attached; failure to attain an important goal; loss of a job; financial reverses; unexpected physical disability; and loss of social status or reputation. If such an event is appraised as a total, irreversible depletion of one's personal domain, it may trigger a depression.

To justify the label, "precipitating event," the experience of loss must have substantial significance to the patient. The precipitating factor, however, is not always a discrete event; insidious stresses such as the gradual withdrawal of affection by a spouse or a chronic discrepancy between goals and achievements may also erode the personal domain sufficiently to set the stage for a depression. The individual, for example, may be continually dissatisfied with his or her performance as a parent, housewife, income producer, student, or creative artist. Moreover, the repeated recognition of a gap between what a person expects and what he receives from an important interpersonal relationship, from his career, or from other activities may topple him into a depression. In brief, the sense of loss may be the result of unrealistically high goals and grandiose expectations.

[1]For a more comprehensive account of the predisposition to depression, see Beck (1967).

Experiences just prior to the onset of depression are often no more severe than those reported by those who do not become depressed. The depression-prone differ in the way they construe a particular deprivation. They attach overgeneralized or extravagant meanings to the loss.

The manner in which traumatic circumstances involving a loss lead to the constellation of depression may be delineated by an illustrative case: a man whose wife has deserted him unexpectedly. The effect of the desertion on the husband may not be predictable. Obviously, not every person deserted by a spouse becomes depressed. Even though he may experience the desertion as a painful loss, he may have other sources of satisfaction—family members and friends—to help fill the void. If the problem were simply a new hiatus in his life, we would expect that, in the course of time, he would be able to sustain his loss without becoming clinically depressed. Nonetheless, we know that certain vulnerable individuals respond to such a loss with a profound psychological disturbance.

The impact of the loss depends, in part, on the kind and intensity of the meanings attached to the key person. The deserting wife has been the hub of shared experiences, fantasies, and expectations. The deserted husband in our example has built a network of positive ideas around his wife, such as "she is part of me"; "she is everything to me"; "I enjoy life because of her"; "she is my mainstay"; "she comforts me when I am down." These positive associations range from realistic to extremely unrealistic or imaginary. The more extreme and rigid these positive concepts, the greater the impact of the loss on the domain.

If the damage to the domain is great enough, it sets off a chain reaction. The positive assets represented by his wife are totally wiped out. The deprivation of such valued attributes as "the only person who can make me happy" or "the essence of my existence" magnifies the impact of the loss and generates further sadness. Consequently, the deserted husband draws extreme, negative conclusions that parallel the extreme positive associations to his wife. He interprets the consequences of the loss as: "I am nothing without her; I can never be happy again"; "I can't go on without her."

The further reverberations of the desertion lead the husband to question his worth: "If I had been a better person, she wouldn't have left me." Further, he foresees other negative consequences of the break-up of the marriage. "All of our friends will go over to her side"; "The children will want to live with her, not me"; "I will go broke trying to maintain two households."

As the chain reaction progresses to a full-blown depression, his self-doubts and gloomy predictions expand into negative generalizations about himself, his world, and his future. He starts to see himself as permanently impoverished in terms of emotional satisfactions, as well as financially. In addition, he exacerbates his suffering by overly dramatizing the event: "It is too much for a person to bear" or, "This is a terrible disaster." Such ideas undermine his ability and motivation to absorb the shock.

The husband divorces himself from activities and goals that formerly gave him satisfaction. He may withdraw his investment in his career goals ("because they are meaningless without my wife"). He is not motivated to work or even to take care of himself ("because it isn't worth the effort"). His distress is aggravated by the physiological concomitants of depression, such as loss of appetite and sleep disturbances. Finally, he thinks of suicide as an escape ("because life is too painful").

Since the chain reaction is circular, the depression becomes progressively worse. The various symptoms—sadness, decreased physical activity, sleep disturbance—feed back into the psychological system. Hence, as he experiences sadness, his pessimism leads him to conclude, "I shall always be sad." This ideation leads to more sadness, which is further interpreted in a negative way. Similarly, he thinks, "I shall never be able to eat again or to sleep again," and concludes that he is deteriorating physically. As he observes the various manifestations of his disorder (decreased productivity, avoidance of responsibility, withdrawal from other people), he becomes increasingly critical of himself. His self-criticisms lead to further sadness; thus, we see a continuing vicious cycle.

The anecdote of a man deserted by his wife illustrates the impact and reverberations of a loss in a vulnerable individual. We can now depart from the particular case in order to establish generalizations about the development of depression. The depressive chain reaction may be triggered by other kinds of losses such as failure at school or on a job. More chronic deprivations, such as disturbance in key interpersonal relations, may also be triggers.

The concept of the depressive chain reaction can be expanded to provide answers to the following problems: Why does the depressed patient have such low self-esteem? Why is he pervasively pessimistic? Why does he berate himself so viciously? Why does he give up? Why does he believe no one can help him?

LOW SELF-ESTEEM AND SELF-CRITICISMS

As the depressed patient reflects about adverse events (such as a separation, rejection, defeat, not measuring up to his expectations), he ponders over what these experiences tell him about himself. He is likely to assign the cause of the adverse event to an heinous defect in himself. The deserted husband concludes, "I have lost her because I am unlovable." This conclusion, of course, is only one of a number of possible explanations, such as basic incompatibility of their personalities, the wife's own problems, or her desire for an adventure related more to thrill-seeking than to a change in her feelings for her husband.

When the patient attributes the cause of the loss to himself, the rift in his domain becomes a chasm: He suffers not only the loss itself but he "discovers" a deficiency in himself. He tends to view this presumed deficiency in greatly exaggerated terms. A woman reacted to desertion by her lover with the thought, "I'm getting old and ugly . . . I must be repulsive-looking." A man who lost his job due to a general decline in the economy thought, "I'm inept . . . I'm too weak to make a living."

By viewing the desertion in terms of his own deficiency, the patient experiences additional morbid symptoms. His conviction of his presumed defects becomes so imperative that it infiltrates his every thought about himself. In the course of time, his picture of his negative attributes expands to the point that it takes over his self-image. When asked to describe himself, he can think only of his "bad" traits. He has great difficulty in shifting his attention to his abilities and achievements and he glosses over or discounts attributes he may have valued highly in the past.

The patient's preoccupation with his presumed deficiency assumes many forms. He appraises each experience in terms of the deficiency. He interprets ambiguous or slightly negatively toned experiences as evidence of this deficiency. For instance, following an argument with her brother, a mildly depressed woman concluded, "I am incapable of being loved and of giving love," and she became more depressed. In reality, she had a number of intimate friends and a loving husband and children. When a friend was too busy to chat with her on the phone, she thought, "She doesn't want to talk to me any more." If her husband came home late from the office, she decided that he was staying away in order to avoid her. When her children were crabby at dinner, she thought, "I have failed them." In reality, there were more plausible explanations for these events, but the patient had difficulty in even considering explanations that did not reflect badly on her.

The tendency to compare oneself with others further lowers self-esteem. Every encounter with another may be turned into a negative self-evaluation. Thus, when talking to other people, the depressed patient thinks, "I'm not a good conversationalist . . . I'm not as interesting as the other people." As he walks down the street, he thinks, "Those people look attractive, but I am unattractive." "I have bad posture and bad breath." He sees a mother with a child and thinks, "She's a much better parent than I am." He observes another patient working industriously in the hospital and thinks, "He's a hard worker; I'm lazy and helpless."

The harshness and inappropriateness of self-reproaches in depression have either been ignored by writers or have stimulated very abstract speculations. Freud postulated that the bereaved patient has a pool of unconscious hostility toward the deceased loved object. Since he cannot allow himself to experience this hostility, the patient directs the anger toward himself and accuses himself of faults that actually are characteristics of the loved object. The concept of inverted rage has remained firmly entrenched in many theories of depression. The convoluted pathway proposed by Freud is so removed from information obtained from patients that it is difficult to test it.

A careful examination of the patient's statements provides a more parsimonious explanation of the self-reproaches. A clue to the genesis of the self-criticisms is found in the observation that many depressed patients are critical of attributes they previously had valued highly. For example, a woman who had enjoyed looking at herself in the mirror berated herself with indignities such as "I'm getting old and ugly." Another acutely depressed woman who had always traded on her conversational ability and had enjoyed the resulting attention castigated herself with the thought, "I've lost my ability to interest people . . . I can't even carry on a decent conversation." In both cases, the depression had been precipitated by disruption of a close interpersonal relationship.

In reviewing the histories of depressed patients, we often find that the patient has counted on the attribute that he now debases for balancing the usual stresses of life, mastering new problems, and attaining important objectives. When he reaches the conclusion (often erroneously) that he is unable to master a serious problem, attain a goal, or forestall a loss, he downgrades the asset.

As this attribute appears to fade, he begins to believe that he cannot get satisfaction out of life and that all he can expect is pain and suffering. The depressed patient proceeds from disappointment to self-blame to pessimism.

To illustrate the mechanism of self-blame, we might consider the sequence in which the average person blames and punishes somebody who has offended him. First, he tries to find some bad trait in the offender to account for his noxious behavior—insensitivity, selfishness, etc. He then generalizes this characteristic flaw to encompass his total image of the offender—"He's a selfish person"; "he's bad." After such a moral judgment, he may consider ways to punish the offender. He not only downgrades the other person, but, given the opportunity, he may strike at some sensitive point in order to hurt him. Finally, because the offender has brought him pain, he may want to sever the relationship, to reject the other person totally.

The self-castigating depressed patient reacts similarly to his own presumed deficiency and makes himself the target of attack. He regards himself at fault and deserving of blame. He goes beyond the Biblical injunction, "If thine eye offends thee, pluck it out." His moral condemnation spreads from the particular trait to the totality of his self-concept, and is often accompanied by feelings of self-revulsion. The ultimate of his self-condemnation is total self-rejection—just as though he were discarding another person.

Consider the effects of self-criticism, self-condemnation, and self-rejection. The patient reacts to his own onslaughts as if they were directed at him by another person: he feels hurt, sad, humiliated.

Freud and many more recent writers have attributed

the sadness to a transformation of anger turned inwards. By a kind of "alchemy," retroflected anger is supposedly converted into depressed feelings. A simpler explanation is that the sadness is the result of the self-instigated lowering of self-esteem. Suppose I inform a student that his performance is inferior and that he accepts the assessment as fair. Even though I communicate my evaluation without anger and may, in fact, express regret or empathy, he is likely to feel sad. The lowering of his self-esteem suffices to make him sad. Similarly, if the student makes a negative evaluation of himself, he feels sad. The depressed patient is like the self-devaluing student; he feels sad because he lowers his sense of worth by his negative evaluations.

When a depressed patient makes a negative evaluation of himself, he generally does not feel angry with himself; in his frame of reference he is simply making an objective judgment. Similarly, he reacts with sadness when he believes that somebody else is devaluating him.

PESSIMISM

Pessimism sweeps like a tidal wave into the thought content of depressed patients. To some degree, we all tend to "live in the future." We interpret experience not only in terms of what the event means right now, but also in terms of its possible consequences. A young man who had just received a compliment from his girl friend looks forward to receiving more compliments; he might think, "she really likes me," and he foresees a more intimate relationship with her. But, if he is disappointed or rejected, he is likely to anticipate a repetition of this type of unpleasant experience.

Depressed patients have a special penchant for expecting future adversities and experiencing them as though they were happening in the present or had already occurred. For example, a man who suffered a mild business reversal began to think in terms of ultimate bankruptcy. As he dwelt on the theme of bankruptcy, he began to regard himself as already bankrupt. Consequently, he started to feel the same degree of sadness as though he had already suffered bankruptcy.

The predictions of depressed patients tend to be overgeneralized and extreme. Since the patients regard the future as an extension of the present, they expect a deprivation or defeat to continue permanently. If a patient feels miserable now, it means he will always feel miserable. The absolute, global pessimism is expressed in statements such as "things won't ever work out for me"; "life is meaningless . . . It's never going to be any different." The depressed patient judges that, since he cannot achieve a major goal now, he never will. He cannot see the possibility of substituting other rewarding goals. Moreover, if a problem appears insoluble now, he assumes he will never be able to find a way of working it out or somehow bypassing it.

Another stream leading to pessimism arises from the patient's negative self-concept. We have noted that the trauma of a loss is especially damaging because it implies to the patient that he is defective in some way. Since he considers the presumed deficiency an integral part of himself, he is likely to regard it as permanent. Nobody else can help restore a lost talent or attribute. Moreover, his pessimistic view leads him to expect his "flaw" to become progressively worse.

Such pessimism is especially likely to strike a person

who generally considers himself instrumental in reaching his major life goals. He characteristically relies on his own ability, personal attractiveness, or vigor to attain his objectives. A depressed writer, for instance, did not receive the degree of praise for one of his works that he had expected. His failure to live up to his expectations led him to two conclusions: first, his writing ability was deteriorating; second, since creative ability is intrinsic, his loss could not be salvaged by anybody else. The loss was, therefore, irreversible.

A similar reaction was reported by a student who was unsuccessful in a competition for an award in mathematics. His reaction was, "I've lost my mathematical ability. . . I'm never going to do well in a competitive situation." Since not winning was tantamount (for him) to complete failure, this meant that his whole life, past, present, and future was a failure.

An energetic career woman who developed transitory back trouble and had to be confined to bed, became depressed. She concluded that she would always be bedridden. She incorrectly regarded her temporary disability as permanent and irremediable.

As pessimism envelops the patient's total failure orientation, his thinking is dominated by ideas such as, "The game is over. . . I don't have a second chance. Life has passed me by. . . It's too late to do anything about it." His losses seem irrevocable; his problems, unsolvable.

Pessimism not only engulfs the distant future, but permeates every wish and every task that the patient undertakes. A housewife, who was listing her domestic duties, automatically predicted before starting each new activity that she would be unable to do it. A depressed physician expected, prior to seeing each new patient, that he would be unable to make a diagnosis.

The negative expectations are so strong that even though the patient may be successful in a specific task (for example, the doctor's making the diagnosis), he expects to fail the very next time. He evidently screens out, or fails to integrate, successful experiences that contradict his negative view of himself.

SNOWBALLING OF SADNESS AND APATHY

Although the onset of depression may be sudden, its full development spreads over a period of days or weeks. The patient experiences a gradual increase in intensity of sadness and of other symptoms until he "hits bottom." Each repetition of the idea of loss is so strong that it constitutes a fresh experience of loss which is added to the previous inventory of perceived losses. With each successive "loss," further sadness is generated.

As described previously (Chapter 4) any psychopathological condition is characterized by sensitivity to particular types of experiences. The depressed person tends to extract elements suggestive of loss and to gloss over other features that are not consonant with, or are contradictory to, this interpretation. As a result of such "selective abstraction," the patient overinterprets daily events in terms of loss and is oblivious to more positive interpretations; he is hypersensitive to stimuli suggestive of loss and is blind to stimuli representing gain. He shows the same type of selectivity in recalling past experiences. He is facile in recalling unpleasant experiences, but may "draw a blank" when questioned about positive experiences. This selectivity in memory has been demonstrated experimentally by Lishman (1972).

As a result of this "tunnel vision," the patient becomes impermeable to stimuli that can arouse pleasant emotions. Although he may be able to acknowledge that certain events are favorable, his attitudes block any happy feelings: "I don't deserve to be happy." "I'm different from other people, and I can't feel happy over the things that make them happy." "How can I be happy when everything else is bad?" Similarly, comical situations do not strike him as funny because of his negative set and his tendency toward self-reference: "There is nothing funny about my life." He has difficulty in experiencing anger because he views himself as responsible for and deserving of any rude or insulting actions of other people.

The tendency to think in absolute terms contributes to the cumulative arousal of sadness. He tends to dwell increasingly on extreme ideas such as "Life is meaningless"; "Nobody loves me"; "I'm totally inadequate"; "I have nothing left."

By downgrading qualities that are closely linked with gratification, the patient takes away gratification from himself. In depreciating his attractiveness, a depressed patient is, in effect, saying, "I no longer can enjoy my physical appearance, or compliments I receive for it, or the friendships that it helped me to form and maintain." The loss of gratification evidently trips a mechanism that reverses the direction of affect arousal—from happiness to sadness. The prevailing tide of pessimism maintains the continual state of sadness.

While the usual consequence of loss is sadness, the passive resignation shown by some depressives may lead to a different emotional state. When the depressed patient regards himself as totally defeated and consequently gives up his goals, he is apt to feel apathetic. Since apathy often is experienced as an absence of feeling, the patient may interpret this state as a sign that he is incapable of emotion, that he is "dead inside."

MOTIVATIONAL CHANGES

The reversals in major objectives are among the most puzzling characteristics of the seriously depressed patient. He not only desires to avoid experiences that formerly gratified him or represented the mainstream of his life, but he is drawn toward a state of inactivity. He even seeks to withdraw from life completely via suicide.

To understand the link between the changes in motivation and the patient's perception of loss, it is valuable to consider the ways in which he has "given up." He no longer feels attracted to the kinds of enterprises he ordinarily would undertake spontaneously. In fact, he finds that he has to force himself to engage in his usual activities. He goes through the motions of attending to his ordinary affairs because he believes he should, or because he knows it is "the right thing to do," because others urge him to do it—but not because he wants to. He finds he has to work against a powerful inner resistance, as though he were trying to drive an automobile with the brakes on or to swim upstream.

In the most extreme cases, the patient experiences "paralysis of the will": He is devoid of spontaneous desire to do anything except to remain in a state of inertia. Nor can he mobilize "will power" to force himself to do what he believes he ought to do.

From this description of the motivational changes, one might surmise that, perhaps, some physically depleting disease has overwhelmed the patient so that he does not have the strength or resources to make even a minimal exertion. An acute or debilitating illness such as pneumonia or advanced cancer would conceivably reduce a person to such a state of immobility. The physical-depletion notion, however, is contradicted by the patient's own observation that he feels a strong drive to *avoid* "constructive" or "normal" activities: His inertia is deceptive in that it is derived not only from a desire to be passive, but also from a less obvious desire to shrink from any situation he regards as unpleasant. He may feel repelled by the thought of performing even elementary functions such as getting out of bed, dressing himself, and attending to personal needs. A retarded, depressed woman would rapidly dive under the bed-covers whenever I entered the room. She would become exceptionally aroused and even energetic in her attempt to escape from an activity that she was pressed to engage in. In contrast, the physically ill person generally wants to be active. It is often necessary to enforce bedrest in order to keep him from taxing himself. The depressed patient's desire to avoid activity and to escape from his current environment are the consequences of his peculiar constructions: the negative view of his future, his environment, and himself.

Everyday experiences—as well as a number of well-designed experiments—demonstrate that when a person believes he cannot succeed at a task, he is likely to give up. He adopts the attitude, "there's no use trying," and does not feel any spontaneous drive to work at it. Moreover, the belief that the task is pointless and that even successful completion is meaningless, minimizes his motivation.

Since the depressed patient expects negative outcomes, he does not experience any internal stimulation to make an effort; he sees no point in trying because he believes the goals are meaningless. People generally try to avoid situations they expect to be painful; because the depressed patient perceives most situations as onerous, boring, or painful, he desires to avoid even the usual amenities of living. These avoidance desires are powerful enough to override any tendencies toward constructive, goal-directed activity.

The setting for the patient's powerful desire to seek a passive state is illustrated by this sequence of thoughts: "I'm too fatigued and sad to do anything. If I am active I shall only feel worse. But if I lie down, I can conserve my strength and my bad feelings will go away." Unfortunately, this attempt to escape from the unpleasant feeling by being passive does not work; if anything, it enhances the dysphoria. The patient finds that far from obtaining any respite from his unpleasant thoughts and feelings, he becomes more preoccupied with them.

SUICIDAL BEHAVIOR

Suicidal wishes and suicide attempts may be regarded as the ultimate expression of the desire to escape. The depressed patient sees his future as filled with suffering. He cannot visualize any way of improving his lot; he does not believe he will get better. On the basis of these premises, suicide seems to be a rational course of action. It not only promises an end to his own misery but presumably will relieve his family of a burden. Once the patient regards death as more desirable than life, he feels attracted to suicide. The more hopeless and painful his life seems, the stronger his desire to end his life.

The wish to find surcease through suicide is illustrated in the lament of a depressed woman who had been rejected by her lover. "There's no sense in living. There's nothing here for me. I need love and I don't have it anymore. I can't be happy without love—only miserable. It will just be the same misery, day in and day out. It's senseless to go on."

The desire to escape from the apparent futility of existence is illustrated by the stream of thought of another depressed patient. "Life means just going through another day. It doesn't make any sense. There's nothing that can give me any satisfaction. The future isn't there—I just don't want life anymore. I want to get out of here. . . It's stupid just to go on living."

Another premise underlying the suicidal wishes is the belief that everybody would be better off if he were dead. Since he regards himself as worthless and as a burden, arguments that his family would be hurt if he died seem hollow to him. How can they be injured by losing a burden? One patient envisioned suicide as doing her parents a favor. She would not only end her own pain, but would relieve them of psychological and financial burdens. "I'm just taking money from my parents. They would use it to better advantage. They wouldn't have to support me. My father wouldn't have to work so hard, and they could travel. I'm unhappy taking their money, and they could be happy with it."

EXPERIMENTAL STUDIES OF DEPRESSION

Although the preceding formulations of depression were derived primarily from clinical observations and reports by depressed patients, it has been possible to subject these hypotheses to a series of correlational and experimental studies. These studies support the model of depression I have presented in this chapter.

DREAMS AND OTHER IDEATIONAL MATERIAL

I observed that depressed patients in psychotherapy showed a higher proportion of dreams with negative outcomes than did a matched group of nondepressed psychiatric patients. A typical dream of a depressed patient showed this content: The dreamer was portrayed as a "loser"; he suffered deprivation of some tangible object, loss of self-esteem, or loss of a person to whom he was attached. Other themes in dreams included the dreamer's being portrayed as inept, repulsive, defective, or thwarted in attempting to reach a goal. This observation was borne out in a systematic study (Beck and Hurvich, 1959).

The theme of deprivation and thwarting are apparent in the following typical dreams of depressed patients: The dreamer desperately wanted to call his wife. He inserted his only coin into a pay telephone. He got the wrong number; since he had wasted his only coin, he was unable to reach his wife and felt sad. Another patient dreamed he was very thirsty. He ordered a glass of beer at a bar. He was served a drink containing a mixture of beer and scotch! He felt disappointed and helpless.

The finding of typical negative themes was validated in a second, more refined study of the most recent dreams of 228 depressed and nondepressed psychiatric patients (Beck and Ward, 1961).

Another approach to the thinking patterns in depression was based on the administration of the Focussed

Fantasy Test. The materials consisted of a set of cards; each card contained four frames depicting a continuous sequence of events involving a set of identical twins. The plot was similar to that observed in dreams of depressed patients; namely, one of the twins loses something of value, is rejected, or punished. Depressed patients were much more likely than nondepressed patients to identify with the twin who was the "loser" in each sequence.

In the long-term clinical study previously noted (Beck, 1963), I analyzed the verbatim recorded verbal productions of 81 depressed and nondepressed patients in psychotherapy. I found that depressed patients distorted their experiences in an idiosyncratic way. They misinterpreted events in terms of deprivation, personal failure, or rejection; or they exaggerated the significance of events that seemed to reflect badly on them. They also perserverated in making indiscriminate, negative predictions. The distorted appraisals of reality showed a similarity to the content of the dreams.

Our research group has conducted a series of correlational studies to test these clinical findings. We found significant correlations between the depth of depression and the degree of pessimism and negative self-evaluations. After recovery from depression, the patients showed a remarkable improvement in their outlook and self-appraisals (Beck, 1972b). These findings lent strong support to the thesis that depression is associated with a negative view of the self and the future. The high correlation between measures of negative view of the future and negative view of the self supported the concept of the cognitive triad in depression.

The relation between negative view of the future and suicidal wishes has been supported by a number of studies. The most crucial study attempted to determine what psychological factor contributed most strongly to the seriousness of a suicide attempt. We found that hopelessness was the best indicator of how serious the person was about terminating his life (Minkoff, Bergman, Beck, and Beck, 1973; Beck, Kovacs, and Weissman, 1975).

Another way to test the primacy of the negative attitudes in depression is to attempt to modify them and observe the effects. If we ameliorate the depressed patient's unrealistically low concept of his capabilities and of his future, then we would expect the secondary symptoms of depression, such as low mood and loss of constructive motivation, to improve accordingly.

When presented with a simple card-sorting task, depressed patients in the psychiatric clinic were significantly more pessimistic about their chances of success than a matched control group of nondepressed patients. In actuality, the depressed patients performed as well as the nondepressed patients. The depressed patients who succeeded in reaching their stated goals were much more optimistic on a second task. Moreover, their performance on the second task was better than that of the nondepressed group (Loeb, Beck, and Diggory, 1971). We repeated this study with depressed and nondepressed patients who had been hospitalized because of their illness. We found that following a successful experience, the depressed patients showed an increase in self-esteem and optimism that spread to attributes not related to the test. Thus, they were more positive about their personal attractiveness, ability to communicate, and social interests; they also saw their future as brighter and had higher expectations of achieving their major objectives in life.

This change in self-appraisal was paralleled by a lifting of their mood (Beck, 1974).

A similar study of 15 depressed inpatients focused on the depressed patients' difficulty in expressing themselves verbally. They were given a graded series of assignments proceeding in a progression from the simplest step (reading a paragraph aloud) to the most difficult. The final assignment, which all the patients were able to master, consisted of improvising a short talk on a selected subject and trying to convince the experimenter of their point of view. Again we found that the successful completion of these assignments led to significant improvements in their general appraisals of themselves and their future. Their mood also improved.

Our finding that the depressed patient is especially sensitive to tangible evidence of successful performance has important implications for psychotherapy. The meaning of the experimental situation, in which the subject receives positive feedback from the experimenter, obviously has a powerful effect on the depressed patient. This tendency to exaggerate the evaluative aspects of situations and to overgeneralize in a *positive* direction after "success" provides guidelines for the therapeutic management of depression.

A SYNTHESIS OF DEPRESSION

We have analyzed the development of depression in terms of a chain reaction initiated by experience connoting loss to the patient. We have noted how the sense of loss pervades the person's view of himself, his world, and his future, and leads to the other phenomena of depression.

The typical losses triggering depression may be obvious and dramatic, such as loss of a spouse, or a series of experiences the patient interprets as diminishing him in a significant way. More subtle kinds of deprivations result from the patient's failure to negotiate a reasonable balance between the emotional investments he makes and the return on the investments. The imbalance may stem from a relative deficiency between the gratifications he receives in proportion to what he gives to others, or from a discrepancy between the demands he makes on himself and what he attains. In short, he experiences an upset in his "give-get balance" (Saul, 1947).

After experiencing loss (either as the result of an actual, obvious event or insidious deprivations) the depression-prone person begins to appraise his experiences in a negative way. He overinterprets his experiences in terms of defeat or deprivation. He regards himself as deficient, inadequate, unworthy, and is prone to attribute unpleasant occurrences to a deficiency in himself. As he looks ahead, he anticipates that his present difficulties or suffering will continue indefinitely. He foresees a life of unremitting hardship, frustration, and deprivation. Since he attributes his difficulties to his own defects, he blames himself and becomes increasingly self-critical. The patient's experiences in living thus activate cognitive patterns revolving around the theme of loss. The various emotional, motivational, behavioral, and vegetative phenomena of depression flow from these negative self-evaluations.

The patient's sadness is an inevitable consequence of his sense of deprivation, pessimism, and self-criticism. Apathy results from giving up completely. His loss of spontaneity, his escapist and avoidance wishes, and his suicidal wishes similarly stem from the way he appraises his life. His hopelessness leads to loss of motivation: Because he expects a negative outcome from any course of action, he loses the internal stimulation to engage in any constructive activity. Moreover, this pessimism leads him ultimately to suicidal wishes.

The various behavioral manifestations of depression, such as inertia, fatigability, agitation, are similarly the outcomes of the negative cognitions. Inertia and passivity are expressions of the patient's loss of spontaneous motivation. His easy fatigability results from his continuous expectations of negative outcomes from whatever he undertakes. Similarly, agitation is related to the thought content. Unlike the retarded patient who passively resigns himself to his "fate," the agitated patient fights desperately to find a way out of his predicament. Since he is unable to grasp a solution, he is driven into frantic motor activity, such as pacing the floor or scratching various parts of his body.

The vegetative signs of depression—loss of appetite, loss of libido, sleep disturbance—appear to be the physiological concomitants of the particular psychological disturbance in depression. The physiological signs of depression may be regarded as analogous to the autonomic nervous system manifestations of anxiety. The specific psychological arousal in depression affects, in particular, appetite, sleep, and sexual drive.

The continuous downward course in depression may be explained in terms of the feedback model. As a result of his negative attitudes, the patient interprets his dysphoria, sense of loss, and physical symptoms in a negative way. His conclusion that he is defective and cannot improve reinforces his negative expectations and negative self-image. Consequently, he feels sadder and more impelled to avoid the "demands" of his environment. Thus, the vicious cycle is perpetrated.

Experimental studies of depression provide leads for therapeutic intervention. By helping the patient to recognize how he consistently distorts his experiences, the therapist may help to alleviate his self-criticalness and pessimism. When these key links in the chain are loosened, the inexorable cycle of depression is interrupted and normal feelings and desires re-emerge. As we shall see in the discussion of other emotional disturbances, the major thrust towards health is achieved by reshaping the patient's erroneous beliefs.

CHAPTER 6

The Alarm Is Worse Than the Fire: Anxiety Neurosis

The problem of anxiety is a nodal point at which the most various and important questions arise, a riddle whose solution would be bound to throw a flood of light upon our whole mental existence—Sigmund Freud

ANXIETY

Anxiety is generally considered not only a universal emotion but a mark of man's humanness. Who has not felt the sharp edge of terror when something precious was suddenly threatened, or unremitting waves of distress while awaiting an unpleasant confrontation? Freud (1915-1917), who probably stimulated more interest in anxiety than any other writer, underscored the generality of this phenomenon.

> I have no need to introduce anxiety itself to you. Every one of us has experienced that sensation, or, to speak more correctly, that affective state, at one time or another on our own account. But I think the question has never been seriously enough raised of

why neurotics in particular suffer from anxiety so much more and so much more strongly than other people [pp. 392-393].

The significance of anxiety in contemporary life has been dramatized by writers such as Albert Camus, who has referred to this period as "the century of fear" (1947), and by W. H. Auden (1947) in his poetic *The Age of Anxiety.* Leonard Bernstein's Second Symphony (1960) as well as a modern ballet by Jerome Robbins (see Mason, 1954) have the same title. Moreover, a popular book about our times is also entitled *The Age of Anxiety* (Glasrud, 1960).

Of course, the concept of anxiety is hardly new; it is reflected in ancient Egyptian hieroglyphics. Writers during medieval times such as the Arab philosopher, Ala ibn Hazm of Cordova, asserted the ubiquitousness of anxiety as a basic condition of human existence (see Kritzeck, 1956).

The permeation of the theme of anxiety in literature, music, art, religion, and philosophy has been well documented by Rollo May (1950) in his book *The Meaning of Anxiety.* The concept of anxiety has attained paramount recognition by psychiatrists and psychologists as an alleged cause as well as a manifestation of neurosis. It has been estimated that over 5,000 articles and books on anxiety have appeared in the psychological and medical literature in the past 20 years (Spielberger, 1972).

THE FUNCTION OF ANXIETY

Biologists, psychologists, and psychiatrists have long attributed a useful function to anxiety. Many writers regard anxiety as an expression of the life-preserving fight-flight reaction and consider it an essential biological mechanism for mobilizing the organism for action in response to danger. Freud (1915-1917), for instance, wrote: "Realistic anxiety strikes us as something very rational and intelligible. We may say of it that it is a reaction to the perception of an external danger—that is, of an injury which is expected and foreseen. It is connected with the flight reflex and it may be regarded as a manifestation of the self-preservative instinct" (pp. 393-394).

A large body of opinion supports Freud's notion that anxiety serves as a signal of danger. Freud (1926) suggests that anxiety is a warning either of an external or an internal danger (for example, the impending breakthrough of a taboo wish). In response to the warning, the individual prepares for action to cope with the external danger or mobilizes psychological defenses to protect himself against the internal danger.

The notion that anxiety is an important stimulus for preparing an individual physically and psychologically to combat a threat deserves reconsideration. What evidence do we have that anxiety is an essential condition for emergency responses rather than an unpleasant distraction? How can we be so confident that anxiety enhances survival? It certainly is possible to think of instances in which a person can prepare for immediate action without preliminary priming by anxiety. An athlete can readily mobilize his resources for a split-second movement to make a net shot or to catch a runner off base. The spur of the competitive situation is sufficient—without the stimulus of anxiety—for the rapid activation of the central nervous system and a subsequent coordinated movement of his body. If a person is capable of emergency responses without anxiety (or anger), why should we expect that he requires anxiety to mobilize him for appropriate action in a situation of danger?

We also know, in fact, that anxiety can interfere with the capacity to deal with danger—and may indeed increase one's vulnerability in a life-threatening situation. We are familiar with instances of "freezing" in the face of a physical threat. We can readily envision how a trapeze performer or a bridge worker might have a serious fall as a result of dizziness and trembling stemming from anxiety. There is also evidence that prolonged anxiety may produce physiological disorders in susceptible individuals (see Chapter 8).

Leventhal (1969) has proposed a "parallel response paradigm" which outlines the sequence of events from danger to action: external threat ⟶ appraisal of threat ⟶ appropriate coping behavior. Anxiety is experienced after the appraisal of threat and is concomitant with, not antecedent to, adaptive behavior; that is, it does not contribute to the adaptive sequence. When anxiety encroaches on coping behavior, it is likely to have a disruptive effect. Perhaps the time has come for those who attribute a useful function to anxiety to generate more powerful arguments to buttress their position.

The notion of purposiveness to anxiety as a catalyst for emergency responses or as an integral part of the mobilization of the survival apparatus raises other questions. Why do we attribute such crucial functions to one emotion (anxiety) but no special adaptive functions to other emotions such as sadness, embarrassment, or joy? Granted that all emotions add dimensions to human experience, nonetheless, at this state of our knowledge, the endowment of anxiety with other wholesome functions seems to be making a virtue of adversity.

The purposiveness of realistic anxiety has also carried over to the concept of neurotic anxiety. Freud (1926) postulates that neurotic anxiety is caused by perception of an *internal* danger from the unconscious impulses. It is aroused by the fear of what would happen should the forces of repression fail to prevent instinctual demands from discharging themselves in impulsive action. If binding of the taboo instinctual energies fails, then these energies themselves would produce anxiety.

The logic of this formulation is questioned by Hoch (1950) who poses the paradox: If "anxiety is a signal that repressed instinctual forces have begun to erupt . . . why should the alarm burn down the house" (p. 108)?

ANXIETY AND FEAR

The definition of fear is often confounded with the definition of anxiety. This overlapping in meaning vitiates the advantages of using two distinct words to designate related but separable phenomena. Freud (1917), for example, wrote about realistic fears and unrealistic fears—calling the latter anxiety. Yet a clear-cut distinction can be made between fear and anxiety without resorting to a specialized technical meaning apart from common usage: Fear is a particular kind of ideation; anxiety is an emotion.

One of the dictionary definitions of fear is ". . . awed recognition of that which may injure, punish, etc." (*Webster's New International Dictionary of the English Language,* 1949). Another dictionary defines fear as "the possibility that something dreaded or unwanted may occur" (*Standard College Dictionary,* 1963). It is significant that the word fear is derived from an Old English word meaning sudden calamity, danger (*Oxford English Dictionary,* 1933).

These definitions emphasize the meaning of fear as appraisal of an actual or potential danger. In this sense, fear represents a cognitive process—as opposed to an emotional reaction. The specific psychological process is the awareness, recognition, anticipation that something undesirable may occur.

Anxiety, on the other hand, is defined as "a tense emotional state . . ." (*Standard College Dictionary,* 1963). This state is characterized by adjectives such as tense, nervous, scared, "shaky inside." The term anxiety is often used by researchers and clinicians to represent a continuum ranging from mild tension at one end to terror at the other.[1]

When a person says "I am nervous" he means that he is experiencing anxiety *right now.* But what does he mean when he says "I have a fear (or am afraid) of thunderstorms"? He is referring to a set of circumstances not currently present but that may occur some time in the future. In this sense, fear represents a predisposition to perceive a specific set of conditions as a threat and to react with anxiety if exposed to these conditions. To indicate the dispositional tendency, the term "latent fear" could be used. By way of analogy, we might say that an apparently solid object is brittle if it is likely to break or crack under mild stress.

When the thunderstorm starts, the fear is activated and the person thinks, "I am afraid the lightning may strike me and kill me!" This statement reveals the essence of fear: the appraisal of potential harm. The concept of danger evolves from the possible consequences of the thunderstorm; namely, the possibility that he may be

[1]For a scholarly review of the derivation and evaluation of the English word "anxiety," see Lewis (1970).

killed. At this point, his fear, which was previously latent (or potential) in clear weather, is activated and anxiety is aroused. He feels shaky, jittery, tense; his pulse races, his heart pounds, and he perspires profusely. Fear is the appraisal of danger; anxiety is the unpleasant feeling state and physiological reaction that occurs when fear is provoked.

When a person says he is afraid of bridges, of tall buildings, or of telephones, what is he telling us? Obviously, he is not afraid of the tangible object or of its accouterments, but of a specific set of circumstances. He is afraid of the *possible consequences* of being on a bridge, making or receiving telephone calls, or being in (or near) a high building. He anticipates that when placed in a particular situation, he will risk personal harm. His fear of bridges reflects his concern over the possibility of his being injured or drowning, either because the bridge might collapse or because he might fall or jump over the railing. His fear of high buildings is based on his concept that he might fall out of the window or that the building might collapse. The noxious element in making telephone calls is being vulnerable to possible social trauma such as "sounding like a fool" to the person at the other end of the line (such a case is described in the chapter on phobias).

Fear is activated as the person gets closer to the threatening situation. Sometimes, he may become fearful simply by talking about the "dangerous" situation—or thinking about it, or imagining it. Dwelling on the fear makes the threatening situation more salient and more imminent; that is, it brings a distant danger into the here-and-now. The threat is no longer experienced as remote in time and space, but the person projects himself into the "dangerous" situation.

The distress (anxiety) elicited by anticipation of physical suffering, such as having an injection, is no different in quality from that produced in anticipation of a psychosocial trauma, such as social humiliation. Most of us have had the experience, for instance, of "pre-examination jitters" or tension prior to speaking or performing before a group. The kinds of physically traumatic situations people commonly encounter include injury, sickness, or death. Common psychosocial fears revolve around the possibility of disapproval, loss of an important relationship, and rejection.

In essence, a person's fear is a particular *concept;* the content of this concept is oriented to the future and refers to the possibility of personal harm. Anxiety is an unpleasant *emotion,* with familiar subjective and physiological correlates.

There are special advantages to this semantic distinction between fear and anxiety. These definitions obviate awkward semantic constructions such as "realistic anxiety," "objective anxiety," "irrational" or "rational anxiety." It is confusing to qualify an emotion or a feeling-state with adjectives that are appropriately applied to ideas or concepts. Could we properly refer to a bellyache as irrational?

On the basis of the suggested definitions, a fear would be labeled objective or realistic if there is a realistic danger; that is, a disinterested observer would label the situation as realistically dangerous. Similarly, the fear (not the anxiety) could be designated as unrealistic. Attributes such as rational or irrational can be readily applied to the concept, fear: The fear is rational if it is based on sensible assumptions, logic and reasoning; it is irrational if based on fallacious assumptions or faulty reasoning.

FUTURE ORIENTATION OF FEAR

If you question a person about his thoughts at the time he feels anxious, it becomes clear that they involve the anticipation of an unpleasant event that may occur in the future. For example, a patient reported the following thoughts in conjunction with spurts of anxiety he had experienced in the course of a week. His employer entered the room and the young man thought, "Maybe he's going to demote me to an inferior job." As he worked along successfully at what he was doing, the patient had the thought, "If I do too good a job, he may really swamp me with work—and I won't be able to handle it." This thought stimulated further anxiety. When he went to see his physician for a routine physical examination, he thought, "He may discover I have some serious disease that I don't know about." Again, anxiety.

Another young man was reflecting about the advisability of asking a girl for a date and had the thought, "She may be nasty and turn me down." Later, he noticed some difficulty in speaking and thought, "I may lose my voice completely." As he prepared himself for an examination, he had the thought, "I might really fail this exam." Each of these thoughts was followed by anxiety. The common denominator of these thoughts is that the dreaded event is perceived as occurring in the future. It may be about to happen, but it has not happened as yet.

Anticipation of physical harm, of course, similarly may evoke anxiety: a driver perceiving he is heading for a collision with another car; a patient awaiting surgery. After the threat passes, the anxiety dissolves.

The future orientation of fear and anxiety may be further illustrated by a commonplace example. Any teacher who has announced an examination that will be decisive in determining students' grades has observed their anxiety accumulate as the time of the examination approached. After the examination is over and the grades have been announced, the class shows a marked reduction of anxiety (although those who have done poorly according to their own standards or aspirations may feel sad, and those who have done well in terms of their own objectives and evaluations may feel happy).

There are apparent exceptions to the principle that anxiety is related to a future event. For example, patients with combat neurosis experience anxiety long after removal from the danger zone. However, when such patients are questioned, it is evident that they intermittently experience a kind of "time regression" wherein they re-experience an event in which danger was imminent.

Similarly, people have reported spurts of anxiety following a near-accident on the highway. Such anxiety is stimulated when the driver thinks about the "near miss" and experiences the recollection as though the episode were currently happening and the danger still present. Others with chronic anxiety following traumatic episodes tend to experience frequent "flashbacks" of the actual experience.

It is clear that the future orientation of fear generally revolves around the theme of suffering. The suffering may be the consequence of anticipated physical pain, or of an expected painful emotional state resulting from psychosocial injury. Common among patients with anxiety neurosis is fear of loss of control leading to feelings of humiliation, embarrassment, sadness. Among these fears are: losing control of one's faculties as in the fear of becoming insane; not being able to function; not attaining crucial objectives; harming others. A fear related to loss of control is fear of nausea and vomiting in public.

A large proportion of anxious patients are concerned about death (Lader and Marks, 1971). Although they do not conceive of death as a state of suffering in itself, the notion of the extinction of the self produces anxiety. Many people consider the cessation of experience the worst catastrophe that can happen. Hence, anticipation of death has great potency. On the other hand, when a person regards death in positive terms, he is not afraid of it. In fact, a depressed, suicidal patient may welcome death as a form of escape from what seems to be an intolerable state.

ANXIETY NEUROSIS

Up to this point, we have been discussing anxiety as an ubiquitous emotion. We realize, however, that anxiety is experienced in a more severe form in psychological disorders such as acute anxiety neurosis or contributes to psychosomatic disorders such as peptic ulcer (see Chapter 8). This raises the question: How do we distinguish pathological states of anxiety from normal anxiety?

Anxiety is generally considered a normal reaction if it is aroused by a present danger and if it dissipates when the danger is no longer present. If the degree of anxiety is greatly disproportionate to the danger or if no objective danger is present, then the reaction is abnormal. Establishing the precise boundary between normal and abnormal anxiety, however, is difficult and depends to a large degree on social norms. If a person, in keeping with the superstitions of his society, is chronically anxious because an enemy has put a curse on him, is he reacting abnormally? Do we label a "green" soldier who becomes panicky on his first combat mission pathologically anxious?

Aside from such borderline problems, we have fairly definite standards for diagnosing anxiety neurosis. Patients with anxiety neurosis show continuous anxiety when there is no apparent or immediate danger. For example, a combat veteran, already returned to civilian life, who experiences continual anxiety and jumps at every loud noise, obviously warrants the diagnosis of anxiety neurosis. (After World War I, such veterans were considered victims of shell-shock.) This diagnosis would be applicable also to a housewife who feels anxious whenever she is alone at home or whenever she is in a social situation. A man who is continually apprehensive about his health—despite innumerable medical examinations indicating he is healthy—has an anxiety neurosis.

Anxiety neuroses may take various forms. Some acute states last several days or weeks. Other episodes may last only a few minutes, but tend to recur frequently. In other cases, chronic anxiety may last months or years. Since these states of anxiety seem to occur in situations in which there is no apparent danger, a number of descriptive terms and explanations have evolved. One of the most common terms applied to such states of anxiety is "free-floating anxiety." As we shall see, the notion of "free floating anxiety" has stimulated a number of disparate theories from various schools of thought.

THE FALLACY OF "FREE-FLOATING ANXIETY"

A patient is brought into the emergency room of a hospital. His features are contorted in terror, his breathing rapid and shallow, his body drenched in sweat. After appropriate examinations and tests exclude physical disease as the cause, the physician stamps the case as acute anxiety neurosis and makes a note on the patient's chart that the patient has "free-floating anxiety." Since, according to the physician's yardstick, there is no objective danger, he relegates the anxiety state to the category of emotional anomalies due to the patient's psyche or, perhaps, to some hidden biochemical factor.

The occurence of anxiety in the absence of any objective danger has led to various hypotheses to explain the mystery of anxiety attacks. Freud (1915-1917) at one point proposed that dammed-up sexual energy was transmuted into anxiety. Later (1926), he postulated an "internal danger": The patient's anxiety was aroused by the threatened breakthrough into consciousness of a forbidden unconscious impulse.

The organic school represented by authorities such as Kraepelin suggested some kind of disorder of the nerves, a thesis that more recent writers have updated into a theory of imbalance of the autonomic nervous system. A few years ago, a biochemical explanation attributing anxiety to excessive lactic acid or deficient calcium in the blood gained considerable popularity (Pitts, 1969), but further studies failed to confirm this theory (Levitt, 1972). The behaviorists believe that, due to some peculiarity in the patient's previous conditioning, he now reacts with anxiety to innocuous stimuli that were once paired with noxious stimuli (see Chapter 7).

The notion of free-floating anxiety has been derived from the viewpoint of the observer, not the afflicted. If we attempt to examine the disorder from the patient's frame of reference, do we get a picture of pure anxiety—

divorced from danger? Quite the contrary. The acutely anxious patient complains to the physician that he has a sense of impending disaster—possibly that he is about to die. In fact, after the medical workup indicates no sign of life-threatening disease, the patient often realizes his fear is groundless and his anxiety subsides.

The fallibility of the concept of free-floating anxiety has also been recognized by Bowlby (1970).

> Unless we know what is or has been going on in our patients' private environments we are in no position to decide "there is no recognizable threat, or the threat is, by reasonable standards, quite out of proportion to the emotion it seemingly evokes."
>
> Clinical experience shows, indeed, that the more we know about natural fear and the more we learn about our patients' personal environments the less do the fears from which they suffer seem to lack a reasonable basis, and the less does anxiety appear free-floating. Were we therefore to confine our usage of the word anxiety to conditions in which threat is absent or judged inadequate, we might well find the word gone quietly out of use [p. 86].

Because the patient's anxiety seems so disproportionate to any possible stress, or life-threatening danger, the examining physician is prone to discount the patient's mumblings about his fear of death. In fact, the diagnostic manual of the American Psychiatric Association (1968) states that the fears are a rationalization, a displacement from "real" fear, or are simply a surface manifestation of the anxiety. This tendency to explain away the patient's manifest fears blinds the clinician to the thinking disorder in acute anxiety states. As a result, the clinician fails to recognize that the fears do seem plausible to the patient. They are based on his overinterpretation of "danger" stimuli, his distortions of the incoming stimuli, and his arbitrary inferences and overgeneralizations (see Chapter 4).

By encouraging the patient to discuss his fears, the examiner uncovers information that makes this mysterious condition quite understandable. From the *patient's* standpoint, the danger is quite real and plausible. What do we learn if we ask the patient what he is afraid of? At first, he may be so concerned with his anxiety, his peculiar feeling states, and his preoccupations, he may find it difficult to focus on the question. With a minimum of introspection, however, it is possible for the patient to provide the pertinent information. Often—but not always—the acutely anxious patient is overwhelmed by thoughts that he is dying. The fear of dying may be triggered by some unexpected or severe physical sensation. The patient interprets the physical distress as a sign of physical disease, becomes anxious, and a chain reaction is set up.

A forty-year-old man was brought into the emergency room of a general hospital in Denver in an acute state of distress. He stated that he had ridden to the top of a ski lift in the mountains a few hours previously and noticed he was short of breath. Following this, he felt very weak, sweated profusely, and thought that he was losing consciousness. A physical examination and an electrocardiogram at the hospital did not reveal any sign of physical abnormality. The patient was told that he was suffering from "an acute anxiety attack" and was given some phenobarbital for sedation.

The patient's severe anxiety continued, however,

and he returned to his home in Philadelphia. When he consulted me the following day, the patient was vague, at first, in attempts to pinpoint the source of his anxiety. When he started to review the recent events, it was relatively easy to piece together pertinent information. He recalled that, when he had reached the top of the ski lift, he noticed he was short of breath (this was probably due to the rarefied atmosphere). He remembered having had the thought that his shortness of breath might be a sign of heart disease. He then thought of his brother who had had shortness of breath and had died of a coronary occlusion a few months previously. As he considered the thought of having a coronary occlusion more seriously, he became increasingly anxious. At this point, he began to feel weak, perspired a great deal, and felt faint. He had interpreted these symptoms as further evidence that he was having a heart attack and was on the verge of death. When examined at the emergency room, he was not reassured by the normal electrocardiogram because he believed "the disease might not have shown up yet on the test."

After we had established that "the free-floating anxiety" had been triggered and was being maintained by a fear of the coronary episode, we were able to deal with the patient's misconception. I explained that his initial shortness of breath was a common physiological reaction to the thin atmosphere in the mountains; his resulting fear of having a heart attack had aroused symptoms of anxiety which he had misinterpreted as a sign of impending death. The patient accepted this explanation as plausible and volunteered his considered opinion that his fear of having a heart attack was a "false alarm." Following this revised interpretation of his experience, his symptoms of anxiety disappeared and he felt "his normal healthy self" again. The rapid disappearance of his symptoms after the cause of his anxiety was explained provided additional evidence to the patient that he was not suffering from an organic disease.

The fears that trigger an acute anxiety attack do not necessarily center around the notion of some physical disaster, but may be concerned with psychosocial adversities.

A college instructor, for instance, came into the emergency room of a hospital because, "I am so panicky, I can't stand it another minute." The physician on duty made the diagnosis of "free-floating anxiety" and referred him for an emergency psychiatric consultation. As the sequence of events just preceding his panic was described, the following picture emerged. A few hours previously, the patient had been preparing to give his first lecture to a large class. He became increasingly anxious as he began to think that he would perform ineptly. As his anxiety increased, his thoughts dwelt on the possibility that he might not be able to prepare the lecture and, furthermore, that he would have a mental block and would be unable to speak to the class. From this point he conjured up a series of catastrophic consequences: he would lose his job; he would be unable to make a living; he would end up on skid row—a social outcast and a disgrace to his family.

By unraveling the thought content that was generating his anxiety, the patient was able to gain more objectivity about his immediate problem. Alternative courses of action—such as telling the chairman of his department of his difficulty—were considered. Also, the probability that he could manage at other types of work, even if he were unsuccessful as a teacher, was discussed. As the patient attached less credence to his fears, his anxiety dissipated and he was able to prepare the lecture and teach his class successfully. A curious footnote to this case is the fact that the following year he was voted the best teacher at the college!

In both cases, the psychological factors involved in producing the anxiety were not elicited by the examining physician. With a minimum of questioning, the psychiatrist was able to ascertain the sequence of events and thought content involved in producing the "free-floating anxiety." In each instance, a fear of disaster—fear of death, in the first case, and fear of total failure as a human being, in the second—was responsible for generating anxiety. As each patient realized that his great fear was a "false alarm" his anxiety receded.

I subsequently started an investigation of acute anxiety attacks. I made arrangements to interview patients who had been diagnosed by the examining physician as having "free-floating anxiety." In 10 consecutive cases, I was able to elicit the kind of thought content described in the two illustrative cases (Beck, 1972a; Beck, Laude, and Bohnert, 1974).

SPIRALING OF FEAR AND ANXIETY

Uncontrolled anxiety is unpleasant, and is in itself a dreaded experience. A person may experience anxiety, for example, prior to making a speech in public or taking an examination because of the threat of humiliation or failure. However, he knows from past experience that he has to contend not only with the possible suffering resulting from inept performance, but also with the period of anxiety prior to and during his "trial." The dread of excruciating anxiety adds to the discomfort directly aroused by the threatening situation.

Accumulations of anxiety may also be found when a person is afraid of social disparagement as a result of openly exhibiting signs that he is frightened. An adult, who was afraid of having a blood test, was especially fearful that his physician would regard his nervousness as a sign that he was weak and neurotic. His primary fear revolved around the pain of being pierced by a needle and the morbid meaning he attached to having blood removed. His secondary fear—of the physician's contempt—was even greater than his fear of the blood test and motivated him to avoid making medical appointments. Once the appointment was made, his anxiety became progressively greater. The more anxiety he felt, the greater the probability he attached to fainting in the doctor's office. This notion produced more anxiety—and the vicious cycle was intensified.

The continuous anxiety cycle may be exacerbated in another way. A businessman was told by an associate that economic conditions in his industry were getting worse. This remark made the patient worry that he would be having serious difficulties. As he viewed the potential problems as more threatening, his confidence in his ability to cope with them was reduced. As his confidence in his own abilities ebbed, the estimated size of the problems increased. Each step of the interaction between his conception of the problem and of his abilities produced more anxiety.

Another factor leading to the spiraling of anxiety is the way the patient interprets his unpleasant affective state of anxiety. His affective response is scanned, interpreted, and given meaning just as with an external stimulus. Since he associates anxiety with danger, he reads his anxiety as a danger signal. Hence, another vicious cycle is set up: Ideation with a threatening content produces anxiety. The feedback of cues of anxiety leads to further anxiety-producing ideation: The patient thinks, "I'm feeling anxious; therefore, the situation must really be threatening."

This phenomenon is illustrated by a patient with attacks of hypoglycemia. The sudden drop in blood sugar produced feelings of faintness and shakiness. She then thought, "I can't handle things" → "I may lose control of myself and jump out of the window or start to scream" → further anxiety. She reacted to the feeling of anxiety with increased belief in her inability to control herself.

THINKING DISORDER IN ANXIETY NEUROSES

We have already noted (Chapter 4) that a thinking disorder is at the core of neuroses. The interference with realistic thinking is readily observed by the anxious patient himself. The characteristic manifestations are:

1. Repetitive thoughts about danger. The patient has continuous verbal or pictorial cognitions about the occurrence of harmful events ("false alarms").

2. Reduced ability to "reason" with the fearful thoughts. The patient may suspect that his anxiety-producing thoughts are not reasonable; however, his capacity for objectively evaluating and reappraising is impaired. Even though he may be able to question the reasonableness of his anxiety-producing thoughts, he believes predominantly in their validity.

3. "Stimulus generalization." The range of anxiety-evoking stimuli increases so that almost any sound, movement, or other environmental change may be perceived as a danger. For example, a woman in an acute anxiety attack had these experiences: She heard the siren of a fire engine and thought, "My house may be on fire." At the same time, she visualized her family trapped at home in the fire. Then she heard an airplane flying overhead and had a pictorial image of herself in the airplane and the airplane's crashing. As she imagined the crash, she experienced anxiety.

Some of the characteristics of anxiety such as blocking on words and interference with short-term recall may be explained superficially in terms of the disruption of voluntary control over focusing attention. When an anxious person has difficulty in concentrating on an immediate task (for example, taking a test, giving a speech), one might conjecture, initially, that attention has become too scattered to remain attached for long to a specific object or subject. Similarly, easy distractibility by irrelevant stimuli could be readily ascribed to the erratic nature of his attention.

On further investigation, however, a more precise way of understanding these phenomena emerges. The patient's problem stems not so much from the mercurial nature of his attention as from the involuntary fixation of his attention. We find that most of the patient's attention is stuck, as it were, on the concept of danger and the perception of "danger signals." This attention-binding is manifested by his involuntary preoccupation with danger, overvigilance for stimuli relevant to danger, and overscanning of his subjective feeling. The amount of attention remaining for focusing on specific tasks, recall, or self-reflection is greatly restricted. In other words, because of the fixation of most of his attention on concepts or stimuli relevant to danger, the patient loses most of his ability to shift his voluntary awareness to other internal processes or external stimuli. This loss of voluntary control over concentration, recall, and reasoning may make the patient believe he is losing his mind—a phenomenon that enhances his anxiety.

The increase of stimuli capable of evoking fearful cognitions is particularly apparent in persons who are "reliving" a particular traumatic situation. A chronically anxious war veteran, who had been diagnosed as having a combat neurosis, would visualize unpleasant images whenever he was exposed to a stimulus he associated with his war experiences. For instance the sound of a car backfiring, any sudden movement, any allusion to fighting he read or heard would trigger off a repetitive fantasy. In the fantasy he would visualize himself lying on the ground and being strafed by enemy airplanes. This fantasy duplicated an actual experience he had during the war.

Similarly, a parking garage attendant suffered from repetitive fantasies after a harrowing incident. While he was backing up an automobile on an upper floor of the garage, the brakes failed and the car broke through a guard rail. The car teetered back and forth on a ledge far above the street for over an hour until the driver was rescued. Following this experience, he continually had visual reproductions of the traumatic episode. During the fantasy he experienced anxiety as intense as felt during the actual event.

Another characteristic of the thinking disorder in anxious patients is the tendency to "catastrophize" (Ellis,

1962). In any situation in which there is any possibility of an unpleasant outcome, the patient dwells on the most extreme negative consequences conceivable. If he is taking an automobile trip, he dwells on the possibility the automobile may crash and he will be killed. If he takes an examination, he thinks he will fail. If he expects to be in a crowd of people, he anticipates losing control of himself and either fainting or screaming insanely.

A characteristic of catastrophizing is that the person equates the hypothesis with a fact. He assumes that a situation in which there is some possibility of harm constitutes a real, highly probable danger. If his girl friend is late for an appointment with him, he thinks she has decided to sever the relationship. A wart means he has cancer; a sudden burst of thunder means he will be struck by lightning; an approaching stranger suggests the possibility that he will be attacked.

Non-anxious people generally adapt (or "habituate") to moderately frightening stimuli with repeated exposures to the stimulus. Highly anxious patients, however, do not adapt, but rather show increments of anxiety with each successive stimulus. Lader, Gelder, and Marks (1967) for instance, presented sequences of sounds to normal and highly anxious patients. They found that both groups reacted initially with increased perspiration (as measured by skin conductance). The normal group accommodated to the stimuli and their physiological responses fell off; the anxious group showed continual increase in sweating, suggesting that their anxiety increased.

The differences in responses to external stimuli may be explained as follows: The normal person is able to determine fairly rapidly that the noxious stimulus is not a signal of a threat. As he is able to label the stimulus as an insignificant sound rather than a danger signal, his anxiety dissolves. In contrast, the anxious patient does not discriminate between safe and not-safe and continues to label the sound as a danger signal. His thinking is dominated by a concept of danger. Once a stimulus has been tagged as a danger signal, the association between the stimulus and the concept "danger" becomes fixed.

We have observed clinically that the average person shows greater confidence and less anxiety as his experience with a stressful situation increases—whether it be public speaking or engagement in combat. The highly anxious person, however, becomes worse with successive confrontations.

The problem of anxiety neurosis may be epitomized metaphorically as an overactive "alarm system." The anxious patient is so keyed to the possibility of harm that he is constantly warning himself about potential dangers. The stream of signals flowing through his internal communication system carries one message: *danger*. Almost any stimulus may be sufficient to trip off the warning system and create "a false alarm." The consequence of the blizzard of "false alarms" is that the patient does experience harm—he is in a constant state of anxiety.

CHAPTER 7

Afraid But Not Afraid: Phobias and Obsessions

> *I saw that all the things I feared, and which feared me had nothing good or bad in them save insofar as the mind was affected by them.*—Spinoza

He felt a wave of dizziness and believed that he was going to pass out. He struggled to maintain his grip on consciousness. At the same time he felt strangely distant—as though this were not he. His belly ached and he wondered whether it would burst. He felt he was going to vomit. He could feel his pulse race and his heart was thumping perceptibly against his chest wall. He tried to breathe deeply but had difficulty in catching his breath. Although his mouth was uncomfortably dry, the rest of his body was wet with sweat. His hands shook uncontrollably and his body swayed. He tried to speak but the words would not form and came out in unintelligible bits. His main thought was that he was about to die.

This description suggests a person in an emergency. He could be ravaged by an actual illness—a heart attack, or perhaps acute appendicitis. Or, he might be facing an external catastrophe that is producing overwhelming anxiety. In actuality, he is a phobic individual who has been forced into a situation he dreads unrealistically. Unraveling the structure of such an exorbitant reaction to a relatively safe situation is intriguing in itself, and also clarifies further the complexities of human behavior.

When it was fashionable to classify phobias on the basis of a feared object or situation, learned physicians coined at least 107 different names (Terhune, 1949). Some of the more exotic are: ailurophobia (cats), anthophobia (flowers), astraphobia (lightning), brontophobia (thunder), mysophobia (dirt or germs), nyctophobia (darkness), and ophidiophobia (snakes). The kinds of objects or situations involved in phobic reactions have changed from one era to the next in much the same way the content of delusions has changed. In the 16th century, for example, phobias centered around demons (demonphobia) and Satan (Satanophobia). When syphilis was a common concern—during the first half of the twentieth century—many people who were familiar with the fact that it was spread only by venereal contact nonetheless avoided dirty objects, handshaking and the like for fear of contracting this disease.

The proliferation of the names of phobias demonstrates that there is almost no limit to the kinds of creatures, objects, or situations that can arouse excessive or inappropriate anxiety. With technological advances, new phobias have appeared—fear of riding in subway cars or elevators, fear of radioactivity from the dials of wristwatches.

Obviously not every fear is a phobia. There is much in our environment that is a source of danger to our health and life. People are killed continually in accidents—from falls, automobile crashes, fires, explosions—or become sick or die from infectious diseases. A person who avoids blasting areas, firetraps, exposed electrical wires, poisonous drugs, tuberculous patients, loaded firearms can hardly be accused of being neurotic. If he is afraid to swim in a rough sea, drink dirty water, or walk through a crime-ridden area at night, he may be commended for his prudence.

Inasmuch as dangers are real and fears are widespread, how do we distinguish between normal fears and phobias? A useful definition of a phobia is offered by a standard dictionary of psychological terms: "Nearly always, excessive fear of some particular type of object or situation; fear that is persistent and without sound grounds, or without grounds accepted as reasonable by the sufferer" (English and English, 1958). A fear based simply on ignorance could not justifiably be classified as phobia. A person may be wary of large, unfamiliar animals or strange mechanical contraptions, for example. Bowlby (1970) considers reactions to the unknown or unfamiliar to be "natural fears."

Important components of a phobia are the urgent desire to avoid the phobic situation and, as the sufferer approaches the situation, the accumulation of increasing anxiety and desire to escape. Frequently, despite considerable inconvenience and restriction of his life, the patient manages to avoid the object of his phobia and consequently is able to lead a relatively calm life. It is significant that even though he openly acknowledges that his phobia is not reasonable, he is not able to erase his fear nor his desire to avoid the phobic situation.

A more comprehensive definition of a phobia than

that suggested in the dictionary is: *fear of a situation that, by social consensus and the person's own intellectual appraisal when away from the situation, is disproportionate to the probability and degree of harm inherent in that situation.* The phobic, consequently, experiences excessive anxiety in such situations and tends to avoid them, and in doing so, substantively restricts his life.

When the patient forces himself (or is forced into) the phobic situation, he may experience the symptoms of an acute anxiety attack: intense anxiety, rapid breathing, palpitations, abdominal pains, difficulty in concentration and recall. Yet some patients find that their distress is milder than they expected—much less than warranted by their degree of avoidance. The discomfort may simply be a "creepy" feeling, as experienced by some people in the presence of insects. Despite their relatively bland response to the phobic situation, the patients may continue to have an extraordinary desire to avoid it. Clearly, experience does not correct the exaggerated fear or the powerful avoidance tendencies.

The Problem of "Objective Danger"

It is sometimes difficult to draw the line between a realistic fear and a phobia. A pilot experienced in flying in combat develops severe anxiety prior to taking off on a relatively safe mission. A veteran bridge worker develops incapacitating anxiety as he approaches the bridge. In these cases, the person has a disabling reaction to an objective danger. On the other hand, consider a person who develops symptoms of anxiety taking a train to work, and subsequently assumes the greater risk of driving on a freeway that has a high accident rate; it is much easier to state he has a phobia—of trains. The greater the anxiety and disability compared to the actual risk, the easier it is to justify applying the term "phobia." We can readily make the diagnosis when the content of the fear is far-fetched. Consider the person who avoids all outdoor activities for fear of sudden electrical storms, the woman who avoids subways and buses for fear of suffocation.

Many people seem able to buffer or to extinguish fears of situations that are obviously dangerous. We are familiar with the relative calm of specialists engaged in hazardous occupations: tightrope walkers, lion tamers, steeplejacks, and mountain climbers. Experimental studies show that sport parachutists have reduced anxiety as they become more experienced (Epstein, 1972). Similarly, "seasoned" troops experience less anxiety in a combat zone than fresh recruits. Psychotherapists can often apply the same principles that govern people's adaptation to highly dangerous situations to help patients terrified by minimally dangerous objects and situations.

In clinical practice, the phobias are usually so well defined that it is rarely necessary to distinguish them from "normal fears." In most cases, a phobic seeks help either because he realizes that he suffers in situations that do not trouble other people or because he can no longer tolerate the restriction on his life occasioned by avoiding such situations. He may develop painful symptoms as the result of new circumstances in his life that force him into situations he had been able to avoid in the past. For example, a medical student with a fear of the sight of blood may experience disabling anxieties when he is required to witness a surgical procedure.

We know that people who are phobic about certain situations are completely comfortable in situations that produce severe anxiety in others. One patient, for instance, who had never had any discomfort in public speaking and relished addressing large audiences had a great dread of being crawled over by cockroaches and other small insects. He felt intensely anxious whenever he was alone in his apartment at night because of his fear of being attacked by insects. This phobia led him to seek professional help.

Dual Belief System

The technical literature contains many assertions that cloud the understanding of phobias. One misleading statement is that the phobic knows there is no danger. For example, Friedman (1959) states that a phobia is a fear "which becomes attached to objects or situations which objectively are not a source of danger—or, more precisely, are known by the individual not to be a source of danger [p. 293]." These assertions make the phobias sound more mysterious than they actually are, raising such questions as: Is it correct to assert that there is *no* source of danger in the phobic situation? When the patient is actually in the phobic situation, is he really *convinced* there is no hazard?

When we examine the content of the phobia, we find that the fear is rarely bizarre or irrational. Consider patients who have phobias of going into water over their heads, eating in strange restaurants, crossing bridges, traveling through tunnels, or riding in elevators. Can it be denied that there is some risk in each of these situations? We know that people do drown and that they die from contaminated food or water. Bridges do collapse, tunnels cave in, and elevators get stuck. The label phobia is warranted only when the person greatly exaggerates the probability of harm and experiences distress disproportionate to the real risk.

Similarly, speaking in public or taking examinations involve risks of psychological injury. It is a fact of life that other people can be cruel and torment one of their fellows who "makes a fool of himself" in public speaking. An examination involves the risk of failure and consequent disapproval, humiliation, anguish. Thus, the phobias that relate to situations where psychosocial harm can occur also contain an element of realistic risk.

When we examine some of the more common phobias we see that many of them incorporate fears that are prevalent among children at various stages of their development. In reviewing the development of phobias, we shall see that many are derived from fears commonly experienced in childhood. Most children learn to cope with the possible danger and thus "outgrow" the fear.

We still have to account for certain types of phobias that obviously do not involve any element of danger to the patient; for example, violent anxiety at the sight of another person injured, bleeding, or undergoing a surgery. These phobias become evident among hospital professionals, such as physicians and nurses, who are forced by circumstances into such situations and cannot use familiar techniques of avoidance. They experience typical symptoms of anxiety as described previously and, although most seem to become hardened in the course of time, there are some who retain the phobia despite repeated exposures.

The answer to the puzzle is found in the observation that such phobics have a high degree of identification with the "victim." The mechanism of identification becomes evident upon questioning: The person is able to recall either visual or sensory imaging or some kind of cognition that indicates he is reacting to the event as though *he* were the victim. A medical student watching an operation had a visual image of himself on the operating table (see Chapter 3). An intern performing a sternal puncture on a patient felt a pain in his own breastbone. A nurse observing a patient bleeding from a laceration thought, "I wonder what it would be like if I were bleeding," and then felt dizzy and faint (just as though she were losing blood).

Other types of phobias are related to the stimulation of a visual fantasy. A man avoided a section of the city in which he had had an automobile accident. Upon inquiring, I learned that whenever he approached that geographical area he would experience a fantasy of the accident and then would suffer acute anxiety. A woman who recoiled at the sight of boats or even pictures of boats was found to have a water phobia. Whenever any stimulus reminded her of being in the water, she had a vivid fantasy of drowning.

Accounts of phobias point to an important characteristic of the phobic patient, namely, that he reacts to the stimulus situation in terms of an inner drama. Thus, when a person with a fear of heights goes to the edge of a cliff, he has images or ideas of falling. He may even begin to feel physical sensations of tilting towards the edge of the cliff, and an observer may notice that he is starting to sway.

At this point, the mystery of phobias may seem to deepen: When he is away from the frightening stimulus, the patient frequently makes statements such as, "I know that there is no real danger. I now know that my fear is silly. . . ." How can we account for the discrepancy in his reactions?

The patient is able to provide the answer. A person

can have totally contradictory concepts or beliefs simultaneously. When the patient is removed from the phobic situation, he holds the concept that it is relatively harmless. He also is generally faintly aware of having the notion that it is dangerous. As he approaches the phobic situation, the idea of its dangerousness becomes progressively greater until it completely dominates his appraisal of the situation. His belief switches from the concept, "It is harmless," to the concept, "It is dangerous."

I have tested this observation many times by asking phobic patients to estimate the probabilities of harm. At a distance from the phobic situation, for example, a patient may state that the possibility of harm is almost zero. As he approaches the situation, the odds change. He goes to 10 percent, to 50 per cent, and finally in the situation, he may believe 100 per cent that harm will occur.

In treating airplane phobias, I have asked patients to write down the probabilities of harm occurring to them. When the patient was not planning a flight in the predictable future, he would feel the chances of the plane's crashing as 1:100,000 or 1:1,000,000. As soon as he decided to make a trip by air, his estimated probabilities of a crash would jump. As the time for the flight approached, the likelihood increased progressively. By the time the airplane took off, he would figure the chances as 50:50. If the trip was bumpy, the odds would switch over to 100:1 in favor of a crash.

On many occasions I have accompanied patients into the phobic situations (for example, going up a staircase, going into the water, or going up in an elevator) and I was able to verify their increasing expectations of harm.

I observed that many of the patients had an experience that simulated what they feared would happen. When I accompanied a woman with a fear of heights to the top of a hill, she started to feel dizzy, began to sway and "felt" a force pulling her over to the edge. On the fortieth floor of a skyscraper, she "felt" the floor tilt to a steep angle. A woman with a fear of water had a visual image of herself drowning, even though she was just on the beach. She started to gasp as though she were actually drowning. A man who was concerned about having a heart attack when he was away from medical help, would feel pains in his chest. Such instances illustrate the phenomenon of somatic imaging, which will be discussed in the next chapter.

It is important to recognize that a strong exposure to the phobic situation, or repeated exposures to a number of different phobic situations, may precipitate an acute anxiety neurosis.

The tendency to have contradictory beliefs about a particular object is most clearly demonstrated in phobias, but is present in the other emotional disorders as well. As in phobias, one of the concepts tends to be relatively primitive and unrealistic; the opposing concept, more mature and realistic. When the unrealistic concept is dominant, then other signs of the neurosis, e.g., emotional distress, are likely to appear.

The Ideational Core of Phobias

What is the phobic patient really afraid of? Since the patient often labels his problem according to the circumstances in which his anxiety occurs, many writers have fallen into a semantic trap. Without questioning him further, they assume that the patient who says he is afraid of crowded places, for example, means that the source of his fear is the situation itself—the crowded place. Since these situations often appear innocuous, such writers have developed convoluted explanations for the fear. The explanations offered by psychoanalysts and behaviorists have several points in common which will be described briefly here.

Behavior therapists assert that the phobic is not primarily afraid of heights, elevators, or horses because of an intrinsic danger in the phobic object. They propose basically an "accidental conditioning" theory of phobias. Wolpe (1969) for instance, postulates that a phobia develops in the following fashion: First, a frightening incident occurs and produces anxiety. Another (neutral) stimulus is present at the time of, or prior to, the frightening event. Second, the neutral stimulus becomes linked to the anxiety through this adventitious association. Thereafter, the person becomes anxious in the presence of the "neutral" stimulus, i.e., he develops a phobia of this stimulus.

Psychoanalysts similarly postulate an indirect connection between the source of the fear and the specific content of the fear that the patient experiences. The individual displaces his "real" fear onto some innocuous external object. As Freud (1933) said "In phobias it is very easy to observe the way in which this internal danger is transformed into an external one" (p. 84). For example, a woman has unconscious prostitution fantasies. Since these taboo fantasies stimulate anxiety, she transforms (displaces) her fear of being a prostitute into a more socially acceptable one; she develops a street phobia (Snaith, 1968).

Part of the reason for the tortuous explanations advanced by other writers seems to be the notion that the patient's fear is so far-fetched that it must be associated with or derived from something else that threatens his safety or values. If you question the patient, however, his fear no longer seems so absurd. An adolescent girl, for example, came to a clinic because she had a fear of eating solid foods. Her parents and pediatrician regarded this fear as absurd and did not attempt to ascertain what she was actually afraid of. In the course of the psychiatric interview, she related that she was afraid of choking to death. She had had an experience of choking on a large piece of meat a few years previously and, unable to catch her breath, believed she would die. Subsequently, she was particularly sensitive to stories of people choking to death—which tended to reinforce her fear. Viewed in this context, her fear is more understandable, and it is not necessary to search for other circuitous explanations. Moreover, it becomes clear that the source of her anxiety is not simply a matter of her eating solid food *per se*, but her expectation of choking.

When patients with other kinds of phobias are questioned carefully, it becomes apparent that they also are afraid not of a particular situation or object in itself, but of the *consequences* of their being in the situation or in contact with the object: A person with a phobia of heights indicates that he is afraid of falling; a person with a phobia of social situations states that he is afraid he will be humiliated or rejected.

There are so many different phobias that it is difficult to classify them. A number of statistical studies of fears and phobias during childhood indicate that they cluster into three major categories: (1) fears based on man-made dangers, such as being attacked, kidnapped, or having an operation; (2) natural and supernatural dangers, such as thunder, lightning, and ghosts; (3) fears reflecting psychosocial stress, such as examinations, fear of making other people angry, and separation from the parents (Miller et al., 1972). The first and third categories are more likely to persist into adulthood than the second. For our present purposes, we shall label the anticipation of bodily damage or death as "physical fears," the anticipation of experiencing psychological hurt (humiliation, disappointment, loneliness, grief) as "psychosocial fears." Many phobias contain elements of fear of both physical and psychosocial harm.

On the basis of 60 phobic patients treated in psychotherapy and a systematic study of patients with phobias by our research group, it has been possible to determine a specific central fear for each phobia (Beck and Rush, 1975). These findings parallel those of other investigators who have attempted to pinpoint the content of the fear through comprehensive interviewing (Feather, 1971). The ideational core of the phobia in each case was exposed through the patient's own report and did not rely on inference or speculation, as in the psychoanalytic model.

It is important to note that although the general nature of specific phobias might seem identical, the central ingredient differed considerably from case to case. Despite such variations, it is useful to specify the most frequent fears at the core of the common phobias seen in clinical practice. The list of specific phobias is by no means exhaustive and is presented primarily to illustrate the ideational core of typical phobias.

Fear of Open Spaces (Agoraphobia)

Westphal (1872) coined the term agoraphobia, which literally means "fear of the marketplace." In his monograph "Die agoraphobie," he describes the following symptoms: ". . . impossibility of walking through certain streets or squares, a possibility of doing so only with the resultant dread of anxiety . . . agony was much increased in those hours when the particular streets dreaded were deserted and the shops closed. The patients experienced great comfort from the companionship of men, or even an inanimate object like a vehicle or a cane." Marks (1969) includes in this syndrome multiple phobias such as fear of fainting in public, of crowded places, large open spaces, and crossing bridges or streets.

When questioned, the person with agoraphobia typically expresses a fear that some calamity will befall him away from the security of his home and that nobody will help him. Consequently, he is comforted by the presence of somebody he knows can obtain aid if he has an acute physical problem. In general, the further the individual is from specific medical assistance, the greater his phobia. Some patients express a fear of intense loneliness or of being lost, as though being alone in a strange place might permanently separate them from their friends and family. Others have a fear of streets crowded with strangers. They fear loss of control, which would lead to social humiliation. The patient may be afraid that he will faint, start shouting insanely, or involuntarily defecate and consequently make a spectacle of himself. The fear of loss of personal control is interwoven with the fear of social disapproval.

Fear of High Places (Acrophobia)

This common phobia becomes apparent when the patient is on a high floor of a building or on a hill or mountain. Many of these patients may also express the fear of being close to the edge of a bridge or of subway tracks. The specific fear is generally concerned with falling and being severely injured or killed. Some patients have visual fantasies of falling; they may even have bodily sensations of falling even though solidly settled in a high place. Others are frightened by thoughts that they might have some perverse uncontrollable wish to jump. Some even experience the feeling of some external force drawing them to the edge of the high place. The feelings of falling or sliding are examples of somatic imaging. Many of the acrophobic patients feel dizzy—which may be either a physiological manifestation of anxiety or an expression of somatic imaging.

Fears of balconies, staircases, and escalators are related to the fear of heights in that the person is concerned that he might fall down. Often the fear is far-fetched because he is protected by a railing or is far enough away from the ledge to make it impossible for him to fall off. A patient with a fear of staircases felt safe when she reached a landing—provided there was not a window nearby. If there was a large window, she would fear falling out.

Fear of Elevators

Although the fear of elevators may seem to be relatively trivial, it may hamper an individual tremendously in this era of high-rise office buildings and apartment houses. Some people are so disabled by their phobia that they are unable to go on an elevator above a certain floor and, thus, their decisions as to where they will work or live and whom they will visit are dictated by this fear. The most common content of this phobia is the fear that the cables will break and the elevator will crash. The person usually has some rough idea as to the number of floors above ground that constitutes a "dangerous" height and will start to feel most anxious when the point is reached (usually either at the second or third floor). Some patients, however, are afraid to travel even above ground level. Others are fearful that the elevator may get stuck between floors or that doors will not open and, consequently they will starve to death. Some patients have the idea that if the elevator gets stuck there will not be enough air and they will suffocate. Such patients generally have other phobias that center around the fear of deprivation of air (e.g., fears of closed spaces, crowds, and tunnels).

The patient may have a combination of a physical fear and a social fear similar to that of people who are afraid of crowds. One patient, for instance, was afraid that he might pass out in the elevator and thus be embarrassed. This fear would appear only when there were other people in the elevator.

Fear of Tunnels

The central fear of traveling through tunnels is similar to that of other closed spaces. There is fear of suffocation for lack of air, or of the tunnel caving in causing the person to be buried alive or killed by the falling structure. Once again, we see that the fear is not irrational, but is improbable. When the patient is traveling through a tunnel (or is in a closed space), he may experience shortness of breath as though his chest is constricted (somatic imaging).

Fear of Airplane Travel

It is a debatable point whether somebody who avoids traveling by airplane necessarily has a phobia. Nonetheless, some people react with such violent anxiety to air travel—even when making a trip to a distant place may be essential for their health—that the term phobia seems appropriate. Although in most cases the person is afraid that the airplane may crash, other kinds of fears may be the basis for the phobia. One woman, for example, was concerned not about the possibility of the airplane crashing, but that something might happen to the air supply in the plane and she would suffocate. Another patient, who was generally concerned about loss of control in social situations, was afraid that he might vomit in the airplane and consequently, would be regarded as weak or inferior.

In a number of instances, I have found that the fear of flying was triggered by an actual traumatic event during an airplane trip. These patients had been able to take flights with reasonable calm until they had a traumatic trip occasioned by bad weather or mechanical difficulties.

Social Phobias

The social phobias represent a caricature of the desirability our society places on being liked and admired and on the undesirability of being unpopular and despised. These social emphases may strait-jacket an individual into conformity with group norms. Fears of unacceptable performance are dramatized by two kinds of situations which practically every student has had to confront. The fear of examinations, technically termed "test anxiety," sometimes produces sufficient distress, disability, and inhibition to be labeled a phobia. The fear of failure can be so intense that the student is unable to exercise voluntary control over certain intellectual functions such as comprehension, recall, and self-expression.

It is interesting to note that when students are informed that their scores on an examination will not be recorded or that they can take the test anonymously, they experience minimal anxiety (Sarason, 1972b). This observation indicates that the student is not afraid of the examination *per se,* but rather of the consequences of a substandard performance.

Public speaking is another bugaboo of students. A typical phobia associated with public speaking is illustrated by the following case: A college student sought psychiatric help because of the intense distress that he would feel for several days or even weeks prior to his having to give a speech before his class. In anticipation of the talk, he would have thoughts such as: "I will do poorly." "I will look awkward." "I won't be able to talk." These thoughts made him feel anxious and also stimulated a desire to get out of the required public speaking assignment. When he was actually engaged in public speaking, he was aware of a constant run of thoughts such as "I look nervous ... They are bored by what I am saying ... They think that I am weak and inferior ...

When this is over, I will never live it down." In view of these continual negative thoughts, it is not surprising that the patient felt tense and weak during his talk and found it difficult to concentrate!

The focus of the social phobias is on issues such as being liked or disliked; accepted, ignored, or rejected; admired or ridiculed. Because of the unpleasant feeling evoked by negative evaluations, the patient is apprehensive of appearing foolish, inept, weak. The kind of situation that will evoke "evaluation apprehension" varies from person to person. Some people have a fear of almost all interpersonal situations in which there is the slightest possibility of being judged. Others may be apprehensive of more specific situations. Whatever the case, it is possible to determine that the person is basically afraid of the reaction of other people to him. For example, a person who had a phobia of social gatherings, and, therefore, avoided parties was very much concerned that he would be regarded as defective, ugly, lacking in social graces.

One rather curious type of social phobia is the fear of loss of control over one's behavior. The patient may be afraid that he will impulsively act in an unacceptable way: He will behave irrationally or start to shout inappropriately. A related phobia is the fear of loss of control over certain physiological functions. The patient is afraid that he might involuntarily vomit, defecate, urinate, or faint in public. As a result, he will avoid situations in which such loss of control seems likely to occur and to be noticed by other people.

The social phobias may be summarized as follows: The patient is afraid that his performance in a given situation will be below the standard others have set or he has set for himself: His substandard performance will be judged negatively. As a consequence, he expects other people to be critical and rejecting of him. Some of the social fears such as test anxiety, may be based to a large extent on the expectation that an imperfect performance will prevent attainment of certain goals such as receiving an award, embarking on a successful career, or being popular.

Multiple Meanings: The Barbershop Phobia

The different meanings of apparently similar symptoms are illustrated by a study of patients with barbershop phobias (Stevenson and Hain, 1967). The authors identified a number of separate fears among patients with a barbershop phobia. One patient, for instance, would run out of the barbershop just before his turn. His basic fear, which was also present in other situations, such as attending church, school auditoriums when large crowds were assembled, etc., had to do with public scrutiny. He was afraid of being embarrassed in any situation in which his behavior was scrutinized.

Another patient could not bear the waiting period involved. He was equally impatient in traffic jams. Some patients are made anxious by confinement in the barber's chair. The essence of their problem is their apprehension of being unable to get away. These patients state they feel like prisoners.

As might be expected, the fear of mutilation by sharp instruments in the barbershop underlies the phobia in some patients. An unusual reaction was described by a patient who was sensitive about blushing when in the barber chair. He was afraid that his blushing would be obvious and make him the object of ridicule.

THE CENTRAL INGREDIENT OF MULTIPLE PHOBIAS

Many patients have a wide variety of phobias, which on the surface appear to have little or no connection with one another. It is possible, however, to find a central theme in these seemingly disparate phobias. This theme generally is concerned with a specific fear of the consequences of being in the apparently dissimilar situations.

A woman had a fear of flying, lying on the beach on a hot day, standing still in crowded places, riding in an open car on a windy day, riding in a closed car, elevators, tunnels, hills, and flying. After determining what the woman was afraid of in each of these situations, it was quite possible to find a common denominator. She had the notion, based on certain superstitions or folklore or actual possibility, that she could *suffocate* under each of these conditions.

The central fear, in this case, was being deprived of air. For example, the feared outcome of being in enclosed places was lack of sufficient air. She had also heard, as a child, that "The wind was strong enough to blow the air out of your mouth." Also, she had been impressed by the notion, "It was so hot, you couldn't breathe." The patient's fear of flying was based on the notion that the pressurized cabin might be punctured accidentally and that there would be a loss of oxygen.

We also discovered she had a latent fear of water, which she managed to handle by always having somebody present when she went swimming. She was afraid that if she went swimming alone, she might drown and there would be no one to save her. This case illustrates one of the major reasons why phobic patients are often so dependent on other people: They require the availability of help should the feared event occur.

Another patient, reported by Feather (1971), was afraid of doors that swing, of driving his car, and of disclosing business secrets. In addition, he had an elaborate ritual regarding taking pills. The striking common element to all his symptoms was the fear that *he would harm other people:* that he might run over a pedestrian with his car, that giving away secret information might have the effect of causing fatal airplane crashes, that the swinging door might hit somebody else, and that he might overlook one of his pills which might then be taken by another patient and cause that patient harm.

Feather also reports the case of a physician who was afraid to travel in an airplane; to sit in an audience at professional meetings, concerts, and lectures; of speaking before groups; and of attending cocktail parties. A possible central theme might be fear of social rejection, but this would not account for his fear of airplanes. The psychiatrist ascertained that the patient, in each of these instances had a fear of *loss of control,* which he fantasied would damage other people. Interestingly, he was not afraid that the plane would crash, but rather that he would go berserk, lose control over himself, and strike out at other passengers. At concerts and similar gatherings, he was afraid he would jump up, wave his arms, and shout obscenities at the audience. He had a recurring fantasy of sitting in the second row at a concert and completely disrupting the performance by vomiting over the man seated in front of him, stepping on people's feet as he left his seat, and distracting everybody from the music.

His fear of public speaking at professional meetings appeared to be related to a fear of demolishing someone else's theory. His anxiety at cocktail parties was related to the thought that he might spill a drink and by the notion that he would impulsively tell people that they were stupid. Again, it is clear that the common theme of the multiple phobias was the fear of harming other people, and secondarily, being embarrassed by his loss of control.

Most people with multiple social phobias are afraid of others' disapproval. A woman was treated for a chief complaint of a telephone answering phobia. She was afraid to answer the telephone irrespective of whether the caller was a friend or a stranger, and she used a variety of maneuvers to avoid answering the telephone. In addition, she was afraid of reading aloud in front of others, making a deposit at a bank, telling stories at social gatherings, ordering food in restaurants, and proofreading typed papers to another secretary in the office.

It was relatively easy to ascertain the common denominator theme of these fears: The patient was afraid of rejection on the basis of her not performing adequately in speech. In fact, the patient had an early history of stuttering and other transient speech difficulties. For instance, she blocked on certain words and had difficulty in reading aloud in high school—but these problems had disappeared. Her fear of rejection was greatest when there was a good deal of possibility of humiliation (Feather, 1971).

These cases illustrate the importance of not making *a priori* judgments regarding the ideational content of phobias. Just as the meaning of a particular phobic object or situation may vary considerably from patient to patient, so a varied assortment of fears experienced by a single patient may have a common underlying meaning.

DIFFERENTIATION OF ANXIETY NEUROSIS FROM PHOBIAS

The consideration of multiple phobias leads naturally to the question of the distinction between phobia and anxiety neurosis. This comparison is important because the patient with multiple phobias may have continual anxiety because he cannot avoid all the phobic situations. A person with a phobia of a particular situation is likely to experience an acute anxiety attack if he is exposed to that situation and cannot escape. This kind of attack is not essentially different from any other acute anxiety attack.

What then is the difference between phobia and anxiety neurosis? Generally, a phobia is highly specific, and the phobic may remain relatively free from anxiety through avoidance. Consider a person with a phobia of being on top of a skyscraper or mountain: He may simply arrange his life pattern so that he is never exposed to these situations.

The patient with anxiety neurosis, however, is not readily able to avoid the noxious stimulus. For instance, his fear may center around the idea of having some serious disease. Consequently, any unusual, unexplainable, or intense bodily sensation constitutes the noxious stimulus he interprets as a sign of serious or fatal illness. Since he is unable to escape from or "avoid" bodily sensations, he will experience anxiety. Often his anxiety produces more bodily feelings, which add fuel to his fear of disease.

Similarly, a person who is afraid that other people will ridicule, humiliate, or physically assault him is prone to constant anxiety in the presence of others. If he isolated himself from other people completely, then he would have a phobia rather than an anxiety neurosis.

The boundary between phobias and anxiety neurosis is sharper in the case of a patient who is "afraid of everything." An example is a person who is afraid of being with people and of being alone, of objects at home and of situations outside of the house. In such a case, it is apparent that the "danger signals" are so active that the anxiety is stimulated continually. Such a patient has a typical anxiety reaction: His thinking is dominated by ideas and fantasies of danger even when he is in a place he considers safe.

DEVELOPMENT OF PHOBIAS

There is a good deal of evidence that phobias of adults fall roughly into two groups: (1) early intense fears common to many or most children which the individual has not "outgrown." These may be labeled "fixation phobias" to indicate that conceptual maturation with respect to this fear was arrested at an early stage in development; (2) "traumatic phobias," similar to traumatic neuroses, in which an unusual, unpleasant or injurious experience sensitizes a person to that particular type of situation. A dramatic example of traumatic phobia is "shell shock" or fear of traveling in a car after an automobile accident.

It should be noted that the ideational content of the fears of the adult patients who come to treatment for specific phobias generally follows the distribution of fears in the population at large (or in a normal control group). As indicated by Snaith's study of phobic patients (1968) the kind of fear reported by his patients appeared in most cases to be an accentuation of a fear experienced by numerous "normal" people in the population at large. He found, for instance, that (aside from agoraphobia) the most common fears reported by his phobic patients included fears of thunderstorms and gales, of animals, of social trauma, of illness, and of danger. The distribution of these fears among his phobic cases loosely paralleled that in his control group of normal people.

In understanding the relation between fears and phobias, it is important to emphasize the difference between the kind of fear many "normal" people experience and a phobia. First, the phobic person regards the noxious stimulus as much more dangerous than do other people. Second, because of the greater hazard that he imputes to the situation or object he experiences much greater anxiety. Third, the phobic patient has a very strong avoidance reaction and generally stays a "safe distance" from the phobic stimulus. Some patients have a "hidden phobia" which becomes manifest when circumstances prevent them from avoiding the phobic object or situation. Then the problems posed by the painful anxiety and the restrictions on his life lead the phobic to seek help.

Early childhood fears tend to center on the danger of physical injury or death. These fears frequently persist throughout life. In addition, older children show concern about social injury, such as rejection (Berecz, 1968).

The mothers of children ranging in age from twenty-three months to six years reported that what their children feared most were (in order of frequency) dogs, doctors, storms, deep water, and darkness. Significantly, there was an obvious tendency for the content of the child's fears to correspond to those of the mother. Moreover, there was a substantial correlation between the total number of children's fears and the total number of their mothers' fears. This suggests a familial pattern—a point we shall come back to when we consider "fixation phobias."

Direct interview (Jersild, Markey, and Jersild, 1960) of 398 children aged five to twelve determined the frequency of fears as follows: supernatural agents (ghosts, witches, corpses, mysterious events)—19.2%; being alone in the dark in a strange place, being lost, and the dangers associated with these situations—14.6%; attack or danger of attack by animals—13.7%; bodily injury, illness, falling, traffic accidents, operations, hurts and pains—12.8% In general, studies have shown that the fears of younger children are concerned primarily with physical harm; older children show, in addition, fears of psychosocial injury such as peer rejection, failure, and ridicule (Miller et al., 1972; Angelino and Shedd, 1953). It should be noted, however, that the children are afraid of these social traumas only if they attach importance to the events—that is, if they are concerned about the consequences, e.g., feelings of sadness, loneliness, embarrassment, guilt, or grief.

It is of considerable importance that the reported fears are related to dangers that actually exist in the environment. Lower-class boys fear switchblades, whippings, robbers, killers, guns, and violence; whereas upper-class boys fear car accidents, getting killed, juvenile delinquents, disaster, and other more nebulous events. Lower-class girls fear animals, strangers, and acts of violence, whereas upper-class girls fear kidnappers, heights, and a variety of other traumatic events not mentioned by lower-class girls, such as train wrecks and shipwrecks.

Fixation phobias are derived from the common childhood fears that the patient apparently does not outgrow and which he acknowledges having had as far back as he can remember. Typical examples are fears of the water, gales and thunderstorms, doctors, blood, etc. In a number of cases in which a young adult patient had a phobia as far back as he could remember, I specifically asked the patient whether his parents had the same phobia or to inquire of his parents whether they had similar phobias. In a group of 12 cases, 5 patients knew for a certainty that a parent had a similar phobia and were able to verify this fact; 7 patients did not know whether any other member of the family had the same phobia and specifically questioned their parents. Three of the 7 found that one of their parents did indeed have a similar fear (of the water, of closed places, of thunderstorms). Thus, 8 out of 12 patients with "lifelong phobias" had a parent with the same phobia.

Why did these particular patients become "fixated" in their phobias whereas other children outgrew the fears? It appears that the fears were reinforced by the parents in these instances and consequently were not mastered. Typically, the patient observed his parent's avoidance and followed the same pattern when frightened. In other instances, an unpleasant event occurred during the period when the child already had a specific fear. For example, a woman with a fear of storms recalled a tremendous and persistent aggravation of the fear after witnessing a young boy struck by lightning (see "traumatic phobias").

Even when a parent did not have this phobia, it

appears that the patient's avoidance plays an important role in sustaining the phobia. He does not master the fear because of avoidance of the frightening event. With each successive avoidance, the phobia becomes more deeply entrenched.

Patients with *traumatic phobias* are usually able to date the onset of the phobia to a specific traumatic event. Circumscribed phobias relevant to physical injury include phobia of dogs after dogbites; of heights after a fall downstairs; of injection after a severe reaction; and of traveling by automobile after an accident.

The onset of physical fears is illustrated by the following cases:

1. An eight-year-old child developed a very strong fear and fainting reaction in relation to hospitals, doctors, and smells of anesthesia after he had had a very serious operation. The fear persisted through his adult years.

2. A woman with a phobia of high places developed her phobia when she fell from a high diving board and injured herself.

3. Numerous patients with fears of driving developed phobias after traumatic episodes in which they were injured or somebody with whom they identified was injured.

4. A number of patients developed phobias when somebody to whom they were close had a fatal disease. This occurred in cases of patients who developed fears of cancer, heart disease, and cerebral hemorrhages.

5. A twenty-three-year-old woman had a disabling fear of thunder and lightning. She became anxious whenever she saw dark clouds. When it started to thunder, she would become terrified and leave what she was

doing—at her job, home, or elsewhere—and would try to hide in a windowless place such as a closet. This phobia started at age eight when she witnessed a young boy struck and killed by lightning.

6. Some interpersonal phobias also develop after a traumatic event. Examples include a patient with a phobia of appearing in public places after he had a dizzy spell and fainted; a fear of vomiting after the patient vomited unexpectedly in a public place; and a lawyer's phobia of appearing in court after he had had a case of intestinal influenza accompanied by diarrhea (his fear was that he might have an involuntary bowel movement in the courtroom and thus destroy his career).

7. Unusual phobias may also be initiated by a traumatic event. A laborer developed a phobia of working on the road after he had been struck by a truck while painting a white line. The phobia spread to a fear of riding a motorcycle or bicycle on any road (Kraft and Al-Issa, 1965a).

A girl developed a persistent heat phobia after she witnessed a fire in which the charred bodies of two children were carried out of a burning house. She developed a fear of washing in warm water and of eating hot foods or drinking hot water. She also was afraid to touch an electric hotplate either in "on" or "off" position and was afraid to use a hot iron (Kraft and Al-Issa, 1965b).

The traumatic phobias illuminate the conceptual processes involved in the formation of fears. As a result of the traumatic experience, the person radically revises his estimate of the dangerous potential of a situation or object: He now conceives as harmful a situation previously regarded as relatively innocuous.

CHAPTER 8

Mind over Body: Psychosomatic Disorders and Hysteria

A bodily disease, which we look upon as whole and entire within itself, may, after all, be but a symptom of some ailment of the spiritual part.—Nathaniel Hawthorne

THE MIND-BODY PROBLEM

When behavioral scientists attempt to theorize about conditions such as psychosomatic disorders and hysteria, they enter the fogbound coastline between organic medicine and psychiatry. They cannot readily bypass such concepts as feelings and imagination and their relation to bodily functions. They find themselves face-to-face with the prickly mind-body problem that has confounded philosophers for ages and still has not been satisfactorily solved.

The hard-headed may banish phenomena such as imagination to the realm of the ethereal: Someone who is paralyzed because of meningitis has a "real" sickness; a person with hysterical paralysis has an "imaginary" affliction. The notion of *real* is regarded as opposite to *imaginary*. Yet, the patient with a paralysis or pain related to his imagination experiences his symptom as just as real as organic disease.

The problem of psychological versus physiological causation becomes even more complex when we consider the etiology of the psychosomatic disorders. In these cases, it is possible to observe a definite lesion, such as a peptic ulcer or dermatitis, or to see evidence of disturbed physiology with apparatus designed to measure changes in blood pressure or heartbeats. Moreover, the investigator can wisely propound that "hyperactivity of the autonomic nervous system" is responsible for the trouble. The visibility and tangibility of the disorder proves that it is indeed real—an opinion dramatized by the knowledge that the ulcer patient may bleed to death. When we question what produces the autonomic hyperactivity, however, and explore the circumstances leading to the disorder, our confidence in exclusively physiological explanations is shaken.

Typically, someone who has experienced the onset or exacerbation of a psychosomatic disorder relates a sequence of emotional upsets to the symptom. The patient states that when he worries about a problem his ulcer "kicks up," or that when he simmers with anger his dermatitis is aggravated. Yet worry and anger cannot be examined in a test tube, weighed on a scale, or measured by a galvanometer. Moreover, in alleviating the symptom, the physician or psychotherapist addresses himself to the nonphysiological factors. He offers the patient suggestions to help reduce worry or anger and later observes healing of the skin or duodenum. Or he prescribes a sedative, and the patient finds that as his anxiety diminishes, his physical symptom improves.

In attempting to explain the neuroses and psychosomatic disorders, the psychologically oriented schools, on the one hand and the organically oriented, on the other, have engaged in long disputes. Which comes first—the psychological phenomenon or the physiological? Many organicists reject the "tender-hearted" notion that such vague entities as emotions, ideas, or mental images can play a causative role. At best, these mental events are accorded a place as epiphenomena—that is, not real phenomena but rather a by-product of physiological activity.

These disorders—hysterical and psychosomatic—have been subjected to the same kinds of formulations presented by philosophers puzzling over the mind-body problem. One philosophical approach, *idealism,* gives total primacy to ideation. *Materialism,* in contrast, asserts that only the body is real; the concept of mind is an invention. *Interactionism* stipulates that mind and body exist, and that each influences the other. The notion that mental and physical processes occur concomitantly without influencing each other has been labelled *parallelism.* Anything that influences the mind is reflected by a parallel influence on the body and vice versa. Gestalt psychology assumes that there is a point-for-point correspondence between conscious experiences and bodily experiences.

In recent years, under the influence of behaviorism, there has been a tendency to ignore the mind-body problem. Some behaviorists, such as Watson (1914), simply exclude thoughts and feelings from psychological inquiry. Others use the semantic device of labeling thoughts and feelings as "behaviors" to be studied as dependent variables but not accorded an independent or primary role. It should also be noted that some philosophers consider the mind-body problem unreal, the result of starting from false assumptions.

Although we cannot attempt to solve the mind-body problem here, we can use the speculative systems to extract the descriptive-explanatory model that best serves our present purposes. It will be apparent from the discussion of psychosomatic disorders and hysteria that an "interaction model" is most useful for understanding these conditions. This model is more adequate than other solutions to the mind-body problem in explaining the clinical observation. In the case examples, only the interaction model can encompass and organize meaningful relations among the data such as emotional arousal, observable physical lesion, improvement of lesion following psychological treatment, and relief of emotional stress by sedative drugs.

Clinicians have described a number of disorders in which psychological factors play an important role in the production of physical disfunction or distress. Sometimes these psychological factors are defined in terms of some event or circumstance that constitutes a stress. The physical disorders which have been closely linked to emotional disturbances may be divided into three groups: (1) Physiological disturbances or structural abnormalities in which psychological and constitutional factors combine to produce the disorder. These psychosomatic disorders[1] include conditions such as duodenal ulcer, pylorospasm and colitis, and some specific forms of disorders in the groups of dermatitis, hypertension, paroxysmal

[1]The term "psychophysiological disorder" is gradually replacing the older term, "psychosomatic disorder."

increases in the heart rate, and headaches. These conditions generally are triggered or aggravated by states of emotional arousal. (2) Primary physical disorders that are exacerbated by psychological processes. This category includes cases of "psychological overlay," such as cardiac invalidism and severe dyspnea based on mild chest pathology. (3) Aberration of sensation or movement, but with no demonstrable tissue pathology or disturbed physiology. This category includes a broad spectrum of conditions ranging from "somatic imaging" and the hysterias to somatic delusions. In many respects, this group is the most intriguing of the entire category of somatic symptoms related to psychological factors.

PSYCHOSOMATIC DISORDERS

Psychosomatic disorders are defined in terms of demonstrable abnormalities in the function or structure of an organ or physiological system of the body: skin, gastrointestinal system, genitourinary system, cardiovascular system, or respiratory system. These systems contain smooth muscles, not under voluntary control, innervated by the autonomic nervous system. However, the musculoskeletal system composed of striated muscles under voluntary control may also be the site of psychophysiological disorders such as headache and backache (American Psychiatric Association, 1968).

During the past 50 years, a number of different interaction models have been proposed to clarify the relation between psychological and physiological factors in the production of psychosomatic disorders. These models have been critically reviewed elsewhere (Mendelson, Hirsch, and Webber, 1956; Beck, 1972a).

The models, in general, are of two types. First,

psychological specificity models: The kind of psychosomatic disorder depends on a specific personality profile, conflict, or attitude. Second, *physiological specificity models:* A particular person will react to a variety of different stresses with the same psychosomatic disorder.

According to an early psychoanalytic view, a particular psychosomatic disease is a specific conversion phenomenon characterized by symptoms that are symbolic representations of drives or ideas. For example, diarrhea was considered a conversion of an infantile drive (Ferenczi, 1926). Garma (1950) asserted that peptic ulcer was symbolic of an aggressive mother which the patient has internalized. He believed that the edges of the ulcer crater represented the jaws of the internalized mother.

A number of psychoanalytic writers have suggested that psychosomatic disorders represent physiological regression to modes of body function characteristic of infancy. Margolin (1953), for example, asserted that there was a direct relation between the degree of physiological and psychological regression. Attributing many medical symptoms to "chronic and localized parasympathetic excitation," Szasz (1952) claimed that such excitation should be considered regressive, since the parasympathetic nervous system develops earlier than the sympathetic.

Flanders Dunbar (1935), one of the pioneers in studying psychosomatic disorders, attacked the conversion theory. She reported statistical evidence that certain psychosomatic diseases were associated with certain personality types. She attributed such disorders as migraine, coronary occlusion, and peptic ulcer to specific personality profiles. However, her concept has been questioned by subsequent research.

Spitz (1951) and Gerard (1953) related certain

psychosomatic diseases of children to the personality of the mother. Gerard, for example, asserted that asthmatic children tended to have "dependent, demanding, ungiving" mothers who were invariably "charming and socially wooing, presenting an external appearance of good adjustment."

Alexander (1950) rejected both the conversion theory and Dunbar's concept of a correlation between personality profile and disease. He attributed psychosomatic disorders to unconscious conflicts: The same person with a sequence of different conflicts would have a corresponding variation in the kind of psychosomatic disorder he experienced. For instance, Alexander regarded the formation of peptic ulcer as a physiological response to a repressed desire for love and help: The deprived stomach was "watering" (with hydrochloric acid) for love. Asthma, he asserted, was a repressed cry for help. Further, spasm of the stomach (cardiospasm) represented an unconscious meaning that could be stated as: "I cannot swallow the situation."

Wolff (1950), an advocate of the physiological specificity model, hypothesized that everyone had a typical, consistent, genetically determined pattern of physical response to stress. The patient's area of sensitivity, however, might not be evident for long periods of time. When he was eventually exposed to sufficient stress, he would experience a disorder dependent on his physiological vulnerability: colitis, migraine, dermatitis, and so on.

Lacey and Lacey (1958) have produced solid evidence regarding the specificity of the physiological response to a variety of stress situations. Each subject showed a tendency to overreact in at least one of his physiological systems. For instance, one might respond to every kind of stress condition with a marked increase in heart rate, but with little change in perspiration; another would respond with marked sweating and only minimal heart-rate change.

PSYCHOLOGICAL STRESS AND PHYSICAL ABNORMALITIES

Since experimental evidence indicates that under stress each individual overreacts in a particular physiological system, it is crucial to define what is meant by "stress," a term borrowed from physics and engineering. Most writers have defined stress in terms of external conditions that presumably produce internal strains that lead to physical disorders. These internal strains are manifested by states of excitation experienced subjectively as anger, anxiety, or euphoria.

Emotional arousal is accompanied by increased activity of the autonomic nervous system. One or more physiological systems or organs may be affected by the autonomic arousal. The system that is activated is not necessarily predictable on the basis of the type of emotion that is aroused (for example, whether it is anxiety or anger), but there appears to be a characteristic reaction for a given individual: Depending on which physiological system is overly reactive, the somatic manifestation may be a lesion or disturbance of the gastrointestinal tract (duodenal ulcer), skin (neurodermatosis), bronchioles (asthma) or cardiovascular system (hypertension or paroxysmal tachycardia).

Although this formulation may appear plausible, it obviously jumps over many links in the chain. To identify these intermediate variables it is necessary to examine the nature of stress and the interaction of cognitive and emotional systems in response to it. Various types of stress-inducing situations have been implicated in the precipitation of psychosomatic disorders.

The first category of stress consists of the kinds of overwhelming situations that occur under battle conditions. Stressful situations such as combat present so powerful and realistic a threat that anxiety is almost inevitable. However, the battle-seasoned soldier generally seems to increase his threshold for anxiety over a period of time, presumably by developing confidence in his ability to cope with the danger and sharpening his discrimination of the life-threatening situations. Nonetheless, it has been found that practically every combatant has a breaking point; for example, it was found during World War II that most airmen developed emotional or psychosomatic symptoms after a certain number of combat missions.

Other less dramatic threats than those of combat are impending academic or business difficulties that may endanger social or economic status, events posing a risk to health or well-being, and danger to important interpersonal relations. Some types of situations are not so obviously stressful—for instance, an environment that makes it difficult for the individual person to formulate a consistent, rational plan for coping with noxious stimuli. An example is a work situation in which upsetting events occur unpredictably. Since the employee cannot demarcate "safe" periods during which he can relax his vigilance, he is apt to experience a continuous subjective state of tension. A secretary, whose boss was highly irascible, could never predict when he might lash out at her. She eventually developed a moderately severe case of colitis. Her condition improved as soon as she changed to a job with a more stable atmosphere. Similarly, a child may be highly stressed by a parent subject to unpredictable mood swings. Escape from these kinds of situations generally alleviates the anxiety and associated psychosomatic disorder. The return to normal, however, may proceed very slowly after prolonged exposure to stress.

The second category of stress includes chronic insidious pressures. The erosion is gradual and results from the cumulative effects of a number of subtle strains, none of which is overwhelming in itself. A long series of adverse conditions such as frustrations, rejection, and fear-inducing situations gradually leads to a high level of emotional arousal and undermines the person's adaptive capacities.

A third kind of stress is highly specific for a given individual: A particular kind of situation (specific stress) impinges on his specific vulnerabilities. Most persons appear to have specific sensitivities and are particularly prone to excessive emotional upsets only in response to events that strike these vulnerable areas. Conditions that do not affect one person may be relatively traumatic to another. One might overreact to rejection, another to arbitrary discipline, and still another to a presumed threat to his health. Which event constitutes a specific stress for a given individual depends on the personal meanings and connotations for that individual (Chapter 3).

One crucial personality characteristic of these patients is found in anxiety-prone or anger-prone patients in general: They tend to conceptualize certain life experiences in an idiosyncratic way. For instance, the person prone to anxiety and psychophysiological disorders structures innocuous events as threatening and magnifies minor threats that are easily coped with into major calamities.

Recent research has attempted to establish the causal relation between stressful situations and psychosomatic disorders. Using a questionnaire of Life Events (Holmes and Rahe, 1967), researchers have shown some objective association between stress and physical disorder. Clinical evidence, however, suggests that stressful life situations, in themselves, are less important in the production of anxiety and physical disorders than the way in which these situations are *perceived.* Those with a high incidence of physical disorders are more prone to regard the same kinds of events as stressful than are individuals less susceptible to physical illness. A study has shown that the former group reacted with more psychological and somatic dysfunction to the perceived challenges (Hinkle et al., 1958).

The complexity of the problem of specifying what conditions constitute stress is illustrated by a study of asthmatic children. When a group of asthmatic children were literally separated from their parents and lived in a motel, they showed great clinical improvement (Sarason, 1972a). When they returned home, the improvement disappeared. Presumably, the mixture of the characteristics of the parent and child produced stress on the child. For other children, separation from parents might be a stressful condition.

THE "INTERNAL STRESSOR"

Until now, we have been discussing stress in terms of external circumstances that produce a strain. But typical psychosomatic disorders may occur when there are no unusual external conditions to account for them. The stress in these cases is generated internally and consists of such psychological phenomena as the demands the person places on himself, his repetitive fears, and his self-reproaches. This self-stressing mechanism may be detected by tapping into the "internal communication system." In some respects it is analogous to Freud's concept of the superego.

Most patients who consult a physician for a psychosomatic disorder do not present any evidence of specific external stress. They frequently appear "nervous" and often acquire the label "neurotic" or "psycho" (first in the physician's eyes and then in their own). The physician often tells them they worry too much and take things too seriously. Such statements, instead of providing insight, generally reinforce the patient's self-concept of being unstable and inferior.

The hard-driving businessman who develops a peptic ulcer provides a stereotypical example of proneness to psychosomatic illness. Although the same psychological configuration may lead to other psychosomatic syndromes such as hypertension or dermatitis, it is useful to consider this case as illustrative of psychosomatic disorders in general. The "executive ulcer" type sets high goals and drives himself and others in order to achieve them. His outward behavior reflects his system of goals and beliefs that lead to a constant state of tension. The momentum behind his work drive is his chronic concern that he will not reach his goals, or that he or his subordinates will make costly errors. He reacts to each new task with strong doubts. He usually exaggerates the importance and the difficulty of the task (faulty cognitive appraisal) and underestimates his capacity to deal with it (also a faulty cognitive appraisal). Not only does he magnify the obstacles to completing a task, but he also exaggerates the ultimate consequences of failure. He may, for example, visualize a chain of events leading to bankruptcy whenever the outcome of a particular financial venture is uncertain. He may, of course, drive himself for reasons other than fear of failure. Someone who operates on the assumption that the only road to happiness is through total success may press himself just as much as the person who is afraid of failure.

Although there may be no objective evidence of pressure from the outside, this patient's occupation is a stress for him because of the way he perceives his work. Because he regards every task as a major confrontation and he is constantly racing to head off some fantasied disaster, he is under continuous stress. The self-imposed psychological stress is accompanied by overloading of one or more of his physiological systems.

Those predisposed to anxiety and psychophysiological disorders not only exaggerate the dire *consequences* of falling short of their goals, but also the *probability* of these consequences occurring. For example, an ulcer-prone student always worried about not completing an assignment by the deadline or not being adequately prepared for an examination. When questioned several weeks prior to an examination, he would estimate his chances of not completing the required reading as 50 per cent. Despite repeated previous successes, his estimation of the probability of not being prepared increased substantially as the time for another examination approached—up to 99 per cent at the start of the test. Concomitantly, his estimate of the negative *consequences* of failing escalated. "They will decide to drop me from the honors program . . . I will be so upset I won't be able to pass any more exams . . . I'll drop out of school and end up in skid row." Since the student had had assignments and examinations throughout his academic career, it is apparent that his fears of being unprepared stemmed primarily from his internal patterns of thinking rather than external stress.

Why some patients such as this student develop psychosomatic symptoms in conjunction with their excessive anxiety whereas others experience chronic anxiety without physical disorders is a matter for further investigation. In any event, it appears clear that their patterns of thinking are similar. Their attention is fixed on fears of inadequate performance or even disaster; they are "chronic worriers." At this state of our knowledge, it seems probable that genetic factors determine whether psychosomatic symptoms will develop in addition to anxiety.

THE PSYCHOPHYSIOLOGICAL CYCLE

In most cases, the genesis and maintenance of psychophysiological disorders depends on the creation of continuous interaction among cognition, emotion, and physical symptoms. This cycle is illustrated by the case of a forty-eight-year-old housewife who reported a previous history of periodic bouts of lower abdominal pain and diarrhea. These episodes had lasted from two weeks to six months and were obviously triggered by external stresses. She had had numerous physical checks (including X-rays) over a period of 30 years and no sign of organic disease was found. The diagnosis was "irritable colon." Her most severe episodes, consisting of severe abdominal pain and bloody diarrhea, started during the terminal illness of her mother when the patient was forty-seven. During this period she experienced anxiety and agitation, and within a few days her intestinal symptoms began. Her X-rays now showed definite ulcerations of the colon. The high level of emotional arousal evidently produced spasms of the bowel with resulting changes in its mucosa.

Since most people are able to endure even such a drastic sequence as the illness and death of a parent without developing a severe psychiatric or psychosomatic disorder, the question may be raised: Why did this patient have such a severe reaction? In this case, as in most cases of psychosomatic disorder, the patient had a psychological (as well as a physiological) predisposition: She recalled that from the time she entered school at age five, she would react to "worrisome situations" with transient episodes of diarrhea. These reactions, however, did not produce any serious distress until the patient was eighteen years old. At that time, her older sister developed (and eventually died from) cancer of the colon. Subsequently, the patient became concerned that she also would die of cancer. She was likely to interpret any physical symptom as indicative of cancer. For example, when she experienced any abdominal distress (even when the cause was obviously due to a prosaic factor such as overeating), she would think, "This is probably cancer." She would feel more abdominal distress and eventually would have diarrhea. Thus, an exacerbation cycle was set up in response to stress: threat → anxiety → spasm of colon → pain → anxiety.

We can understand the sequence leading to the development of mild ulcerative colitis in this case. Her mother's illness was a stress to this patient in that it constantly aroused ideation regarding the threat to her mother's life (The patient also experienced a revival of fears of her own death). The unmitigated threat led to anxiety and its physiological manifestations. Because the patient's lower intestinal tract was the target area, the overactive autonomic nervous system produced cramps and diarrhea. The sensory data from the bowel were also subjected to appraisal: She interpreted the sensations as signs of cancer and thus experienced aggravation of her anxiety and intestinal disease.

PHYSICAL DISORDERS WITH "PSYCHOLOGICAL OVERLAY"

Numerous patients have a proven organic disease, but because of psychological factors the disability or suffering is greatly disproportionate to the actual organic disorder. In fact, the disability and stress due to the psychological factors may be the sole reason for medical intervention. Many cases of "cardiac invalidism" fall into this category. For instance, a patient who has had some physical disorder of the heart may be in constant dread of dying even when free of physical discomfort or any residual heart disease. He may be afraid to maneuver or exert himself in any way lest he precipitate a heart attack or some other form of acute, sudden death. As a result, he may greatly restrict his activities. The combination of deprivation of his usual sources of satisfactions and the unpleasantness of chronic anxiety may lead to depression.

A case in which psychological factors contributed substantial distress and disability as a result of a pre-existing organic disease was reported by Katcher (1969). A forty-year-old man had experienced attacks of angina pectoris for many years. Electrocardiagrams showed typical evidence of coronary artery disease: depression of the ST segment which was aggravated after exercise.

The patient was so immobilized by his angina that

he was hardly able to walk more than a few steps without experiencing severe chest pain. If he did not stop to rest, he would experience repeated chest pain and subsequent dread of a coronary episode.

The psychiatrist used a combination of behavior therapy and cognitive therapy in treating this patient. By emphasizing the statistical evidence that gradual exercise was beneficial in such cases and avoidance of exercise was detrimental, he tried to undercut the patient's belief that exercise would precipitate an attack of myocardial infarction.

The patient was then given a graded schedule of exercises. He would walk a certain distance until he had actual pain, at which point he would stop. This distance was gradually extended until the patient could walk *ad libitum* without experiencing any chest pain. Whenever he felt frightened, he repeated the dictum: "Exercise is good." This self-reassurance not only allayed his anxiety but increased his motivation to continue walking.

After the training period was completed, the cardiogram was repeated. Although the ST segment was still depressed during rest, there was no additional depression of the ST segment after exercise!

The psychological overlay may be explained as follows: After the first anginal symptoms, the patient anticipated sudden death as a result of a myocardial infarction. He automatically associated exercise with the precipitation of a heart attack; thus, he felt threatened by any physical exertion. The arousal of anxiety prior to walking increased his heart rate and other autonomic responses, which in turn put increased strain on the heart and increased the coronary insufficiency. Consequently, after taking a few steps, he indeed had angina: a classic example of a self-fulfilling prophecy.

Once convinced that the angina was precipitated by his anxiety and was not a necessary consequence of exercise, he was able to progress on the exercise regimen until he became symptom-free.

Another group of physical disorders with psychological overlay is lung disease. Such patients may be conscious of every breath, every movement of the chest. Because of their known lung pathology, they often believe it is necessary for their survival to make a voluntary effort to suck breath in and push it out.

A systematic study of cases with chronic difficulty in breathing (Dudley, Martin, and Holmes, 1964) demonstrates this kind of problem. Of 20 subjects, most of whom had pulmonary tuberculosis or other diseases causing obstruction of the airway, the researchers found that feelings of shortness of breath had no relation to objective interference in pulmonary function. When patients were angry or anxious in response to naturally occurring adverse life situations, they tended to show hyperventilation and dyspnea. There was no relation between actual dysfunction and breathing difficulty. This study indicated that *dypsnea depended on the perception of signals arising from the pulmonary system.* These patients were hypersensitive to changes in the cardiopulmonary system which other people normally experience but disregard. For the patients, however, respiratory change was associated with a threat to life, which was reflected in the subjective feeling of distress. A vicious cycle was set up: anxiety → hyperventilation and hyperpnea → dyspnea → anxiety.

SOMATIC IMAGING

We have already alluded to the phenomenon of somatic imaging in our discussion of phobias. Patients with fear of heights, for instance, often have the sensation of tipping or falling when they are near the edge of a high place and may experience the sensation of being drawn to the edge. A patient with a fear of the water felt as though she were drowning when she had a visual fantasy of being in the water. Similarly, many people experience vicarious pain when they see another person injured; they react as though they themselves had been injured.

In the discussion in Chapter 3, I included the person's opinion of himself as well as his tangible belongings and more abstract values as an integral component of the personal domain. Another essential component of the self-concept is the "bodily self," "somatic self," or "body image" (Epstein, 1973). The individual's conception of his somatic self at a particular time may dictate whether he feels pleased or pained, strong or weak, energetic or listless. His conception of his bodily state may be more crucial than his actual physical condition in determining feelings and sensations.

Visual stimulation may affect the body image and thus lead to a wide variety of physical sensations. For instance, motion pictures projected on a curved screen (e.g., "Cinerama") can create the illusion that the viewer is riding on a fast-moving vehicle such as a bobsled or is falling through space. He experiences the same sensations as though he were in reality traveling or falling. Similarly, motion pictures of other people being mutilated may induce feelings of pain and anxiety in the viewer. This phenomenon of bodily sensations produced by visual illusions is another example of somatic imaging.

Somatic imaging, of course, can occur without visual stimulation. The prevalence of sensory imaging was documented over 100 years ago by Sir Francis Galton (1883). Some of Galton's subjects experienced somatic sensations so vividly that they were often uncertain whether their sensation was based on imagination or actual physical stimulation.

Fantasies or daydreams (without any external visual stimuli) may also lead to intense sensation in the body. Psychiatric patients often describe this kind of somatic imaging. One patient for instance, had repeated, though brief, images of his penis being damaged. For instance, if he heard a window close, he would visualize the window being slammed down on his penis and feel a crushing sensation on his penis. If he unexpectedly saw a sharp knife, he imagined the knife cutting his penis and simultaneously would experience a sharp pain in his penis.

The *thought* of a physical injury may produce somatic sensations. A young adolescent reacted with anxiety to the sight of blood or of a physical deformity. He was particularly sensitive to any stimulus that suggested bones breaking. When his therapist showed him a bone, he thought, "My leg could be broken" and felt pain in his leg and the sensation of the bone protruding through the skin of his leg. Another patient experienced a remarkable *identification* with the suffering or disabled. For instance, when he read an account of a disturbed patient whose arms were pinned down by an attendant, he felt strong pressure in his arms, as though they were being gripped. At another time, he experienced transient dimming of his vision when he read about a patient who gradually went blind. In this case, the idea rather than a visual fantasy, produced unpleasant sensations.

HYSTERIA

Hysteria is a pathological extension of the process of somatic imaging. The most common forms of hysteria seen nowadays consist of some kind of physical dysfunction which is not based on any demonstrable organic disease or physiological abnormality. The bodily ailment may be loss of power in a limb (paralysis, or weakness); loss of sensation in some part of the body; sensation of pain in the absence of any stimulation of the pain receptors; and overactivity of muscles, such as in hysterical choking or pseudoepilepsy.

In examining a patient with hysteria the physician is often able to establish that the pattern of the hysterical symptom conforms not to the actual anatomy of the body but to the individual's conception of the manifestations of a physical disorder. Thus, following an injury to his leg or his forearm, a hysterical patient may have a "stocking-glove" anesthesia—a distribution of sensory loss that cannot possibly be produced by any lesion. Similarily, if he believes that his brain has been damaged, he may experience paralysis of a limb on the *same side* as the presumed damage, whereas the anatomy of the nervous system would dictate that the paralysis should be on the opposite side. The power of the mental conceptions is illustrated by the following cases:

A patient had apparently suffered organic brain damage following a myocardial infarction (Stein et al., 1969). Psychological testing revealed deficits in immediate recall and inability to concentrate. In the course of psychotherapy, questioning by the therapist revealed that the patient had a cognitive distortion regarding the effects of his heart attack. He believed that there was "an artery to the brain" arising directly from the heart at the point of his myocardial infarction. According to his belief, this artery had become occluded, resulting in irreversible damage to the brain. When the therapist was able to demonstrate to the patient through *drawing an anatomical diagram* that his conclusion was erroneous, the symptoms of organic brain damage cleared up.

Charcot treated numerous cases of hysteria with hypnosis. The following cases cited by him (1890) demonstrate that the motor and sensory symptoms were manifestations of the patients' incorrect conception of organic pathology.

A patient was struck by a carriage, which then passed over him. He believed erroneously that the carriage had run over and crushed both legs. He subsequently developed hysterical paralysis of both legs.

In other cases, the hysterical symptom was based on an incorrect "diagnosis" by the patient of the effects of an actual lesion.

A soldier sustained a bullet wound in his leg and subsequently developed a "stocking" anesthesia: He believed the bullet had severed a nerve in his leg. As soon as the physician demonstrated to him that the nerve was intact, his anesthesia disappeared.

These examples suggest that hysteria is the illustration *par excellence* of the phenomenon of cognitive distortion in psychiatric disorders. The patient believes he has a particular disorder of the body and therefore experiences the manifestation of the supposed disorder:

He is unable to lift his leg, he loses sensation in part of his body, his vision or hearing is impaired. When the incorrect belief is modified through suggestion, hypnosis, demonstration, or cognitive therapy, the symptom clears up.

A number of physicians in the nineteenth century suggested that the hysterical patient had a false conception that was expressed in his somatic disorder. The English physician, Reynolds (1869), described certain paralyses which were derived from incorrect ideas. Charcot, however, is generally credited with having extended and publicized this observation. One of the greatest neurologists of his era, he was constantly forced to separate syndromes simulating organic disorders from those originating in a lesion of the nervous system. As a result of hypnotizing his patients, he concluded that the symptoms of hysteria resulted from a "pathogenic idea." This false idea, based on an erroneous assumption, evidently vanished when the hysterical symptom was removed by hypnosis. Charcot's demonstration that physical disorders could be the consequence of psychological processes provided Freud with a stimulus for applying psychological therapy to the neuroses.

One of the most significant features of Charcot's work was induction of paralysis in experimental subjects through hypnosis. The idea, "my right hand is paralyzed," produced the same clinical syndrome observed in spontaneous hysterical paralyses. Some regard this linkage of clinical and experimental phenomena as comparable to the reproduction of human and animal disease in the laboratories of Pasteur and Koch. Havens (1966) states, "In the psychiatric instance the etiological agent was not a cholera vibrio or tubercle bacillus, but an idea, a suggestion . . ." (p. 510).

Freud, having spent some time observing Charcot at work, applied hypnosis to the treatment of hysteria. Later he substituted the technique of free association for hypnosis. This change in approach also signaled the change of focus from the objective neurological examination to concern with the patient's ideas, fantasies, emotions, wishes, and dreams—the stock-in-trade of modern psychodynamic psychotherapists. Freud proceeded far beyond Charcot's simple concept that hysterical symptoms result from false ideas, and developed an elaborate theory. Freud's thesis that unconscious sexual wishes are "converted" into hysterical symptoms, replaced Charcot's notion, and is dominant in the generally accepted concept of hysteria today. In fact, in 1952, the official nomenclature of the American Psychiatric Association substituted the term "conversion reaction" (derived from Freud's concept of conversion) for hysteria. American textbooks of psychiatry have generally accepted Freud's concept of hysteria.

Despite the apparent obsolescence of Charcot's notion of the *pathogenic idea* as a dominant factor in hysteria, his formulation certainly seems to fit the clinical data derived from systematic interviewing of patients with hysteria. The development of the hysterical symptoms is usually intelligible when the patient's experiences and their special meanings are explored. Exposure of the patient's erroneous ideas provides an explanation of the presence of the symptom. The essential principle is that the hysteria simulates an organic disorder not because the patient wants to simulate a disease, but because of his erroneous belief.

Many patients with hysterical symptoms identify with some other person who currently has or has had a physical or psychogenic disorder similar to the hysterical symptoms. The clue to the presence of this particular mechanism of symptom formation was uncovered by the observation of imitative tendencies of hysterics on the wards of the Salpêtrière, where Charcot worked. Janet, one of Charcot's students, later stated that many of Charcot's cases had "learned" their hysteria within the clinic. By observing cases of true epilepsy, and even assisting in the management of these cases, patients developed hysterical epilepsy at a later date (Havens, 1966).

This kind of identification is reminiscent of the "contagiousness" of convulsive fits as manifested by the spreading of the phenomenon from one person to another. Our modern enlightened view attributes the phenomenon to psychological factors rather than to demoniacal possession and witchcraft as was once believed.

A number of patients with hysterical seizures have reported contact with a relative who had epileptic seizures. Patients with other kinds of hysterical symptoms have recalled having been very much impressed by observing or reading about another person with a similar symptom. A patient with a "cardiac neurosis," for instance, observed her mother's progressive heart failure for many years. Her mother finally died at the age of thirty-two as a result of her heart ailment. The patient recalled having had the repeated thought that when she reached her mother's age, she too would develop heart disease. When she was 28 years old, she began to experience pains in her chest, easy fatigability, and shortness of breath—just as her mother had. Although repeated medical examinations revealed no objective evidence of any heart disease, these symptoms continued for the next ten years and led to continual distress and severe restriction of her activities. The hysterical symptoms finally cleared up after combined cognitive and behavioral therapy.

Similarly, a number of cases of hysterical spells of choking were traced to the patient's having, at a relatively young age, read or heard about another person choking to death on food. The patients recalled having the thought, "This could happen to me." Later, while under stress, the patient would become aware of tightening in his throat, especially when eating. He would then think, "This is a sign that I shall not be able to swallow the food properly." The more credence he gave to this idea, the more difficulty he would have in swallowing. The increased difficulty in swallowing reinforced his belief that something was wrong with his throat muscles and that he would choke to death.

The development of a hysterical symptom can now be summarized. As a result of an injury to himself or identification with a constellation of symptoms in others, the hysteric comes to believe that he has a physical disorder. As he thinks about having a disorder, he experiences physical sensations—somatic imaging. A circular mechanism is set up. The person "reads" his physical sensations as evidence that he has the disorder. His belief becomes consolidated, and the physical manifestations are proportionately intensified.

The therapeutic approach to hysterical symptoms depends on the reversal of the vicious cycle. The therapist can demonstrate to the patient that he has not lost control—that he is, for example, able to move the paralyzed limb. This demonstration, whether it be by suggestion, persuasion, or hypnosis, tends to undermine the faulty belief. Furthermore, by stimulating the patient to *image* himself moving the limb, the therapist puts imagination to constructive use. Similarly, the therapist may start by questioning the patient's misconceptions and re-educating him (as in the case of the man with symptoms simulating intellectual deterioration following a coronary thrombosis). As the faulty "pathogenic idea" is shaken, the symptom diminishes, and so serves as further evidence to the patient that his belief in his pathology is erroneous, thus promoting further relief of the symptom.

In this manner, the treatment of hysteria exploits the patient's imagination in a constructive way and produces relief by "imaging away" the symptom. Further, the reversal of the exacerbation cycle, as in the case of psychosomatic disorders, elicits progressive improvement. The essence of the treatment of hysteria consists of changing an incorrect belief to a correct one. In this respect, the mechanism of improvement is basically the same as that in depression, anxiety states, and phobias: rectify the false belief and you alleviate the symptom.

CHAPTER 9

Principles of Cognitive Therapy

> *If we wish to change the sentiments it is necessary before all to modify the idea which has produced [them], and to recognize either that it is not correct in itself or that it does not touch our interests.*—Paul Dubois

We have seen that the common psychological disorders center around certain aberrations in thinking. The challenge to psychotherapy is to offer the patient effective techniques for overcoming his blindspots, his blurred perceptions, and his self-deceptions. A promising lead is provided by the observation that a person responds realistically and effectively to situations not related to his neurosis. His judgments and behavior in areas of experience beyond the boundaries of his specific vulnerability often reflect a high level of functioning. Furthermore, prior to the onset of illness, the neurotic frequently shows adequate development of his conceptual tools for dealing with the problems of living.

Psychological skills (integrating, labeling, and interpreting experience) can be applied to correcting the psychological aberrations. Since the central psychological *problem* and the psychological *remedy* are both concerned with the patient's thinking (or cognitions), we call this form of help cognitive therapy.

In the broadest sense, cognitive therapy consists of all the approaches that alleviate psychological distress through the medium of correcting faulty conceptions and self-signals. The emphasis on thinking, however, should not obscure the importance of the emotional reactions which are generally the immediate source of distress. It simply means that we get to the person's emotions through his cognitions. By correcting erroneous beliefs, we can damp down or alter excessive, inappropriate emotional reactions.

Many methods of helping a patient make more realistic appraisals of himself and his world are available. The "intellectual" approach consists of identifying the misconceptions, testing their validity, and substituting more appropriate concepts. Often the need for broad attitudinal change emerges with the patient's recognition that the rules he has relied on to guide his thinking and behavior have served to deceive and to defeat him.

The "experiential" approach exposes the patient to experiences that are in themselves powerful enough to change misconceptions. The interactions with other people in certain organized situations, such as encounter groups or conventional psychotherapy, may help a person to perceive others more realistically and consequently to modify his inappropriate maladaptive responses to them. In encounter groups, the interpersonal experiences may cut through maladaptive attitudes blocking the expression of intimate feelings. Similarly, a patient, in response to his psychotherapist's warmth and acceptance, often modifies his stereotyped conception of authority figures. Such a change has been labeled "corrective emotional experience" (Alexander, 1950). Sometimes the effectiveness of psychotherapy is implemented by motivating a patient to enter situations he had previously avoided because of his misconceptions.

The "behavioral" approach encourages the development of specific forms of behavior that lead to more general changes in the way the patient views himself and the real world. Practicing techniques for dealing with people who frighten him, as in "assertive training," not only enables him to regard other people more realistically but enhances his self-confidence.

If neurosis is the outcropping of the patient's maladaptive attitudes, why can't he change these attitudes through life experience or through the help of parents or friends? Why does he need a professional helper? Obviously, in many cases the troubled person works out his problems by himself or with the help of a "wise, old neighbor." Many people improvise quite independently—and successfully—the kinds of techniques that are the stock-in-trade of behavior therapists by gradually exposing themselves to frightening situations or imagining themselves in these situations ("systematic desensitization"), or through patterning their behavior after others ("modeling"). Others tap the "folk wisdom," the cumulative experience of their cultural group, through the advice or suggestions of friends or relatives.

Those who come to the professional helper, and inadvertently acquire the label of patient or client, are drawn from the residue who have failed to master their problems. Perhaps their reactions to their problems are too acute or too severe to respond to usual life experiences or self-help. The patient may have been too fragile to develop coping techniques, or his problems may have been too deeply ingrained. In some cases, the troubled person becomes a patient simply because he received and followed "bad advice" or because no assistance was available from nonprofessional sources. And, while the folk wisdom is often helpful and is probably at the core of much psychotherapy, it often is blended with myths, superstitions, and misconceptions that aggravate an unrealistic orientation. Moreover, many people are not motivated to engage in a "self-improvement" program unless it is instigated in a professional setting.

In any event, psychotherapy can have the greatest impact on problems because of the considerable authority attributed to the therapist, his ability to pinpoint the problems, and his skill in providing an appropriate systematic set of procedures.

TARGETS OF COGNITIVE THERAPY

Cognitive techniques are most appropriate for people who have the capacity for introspection and for reflecting about their own thoughts and fantasies. This approach is essentially an extension and a refinement of what people have done to varying degrees since the early stages of their intellectual development. The particular techniques such as labeling objects and situations, setting up hypotheses, and weeding out and testing the hypotheses are based on skills that people apply automatically without being cognizant of the operations involved.

This kind of intellectual function is analogous to the

formation of speech in which rules of pronunciation and grammatical construction are applied without consciousness of the rules or of their application. When an adult has to correct a speech disorder or attempts to learn a new language, then he has to concentrate on the formation of words and sentences. Similarly, when he has a problem in interpreting certain aspects of reality, it may be useful for him to focus on the rules he applies in making judgments. In examining a problem area, he finds that the rule is incorrect or that he has been applying it incorrectly.

Since making the incorrect judgments has probably become a deeply ingrained habit, which he may not be conscious of, several steps are required to correct it. First, he has to become aware of what he is thinking. Second, he needs to recognize what thoughts are awry. Then he has to substitute accurate for inaccurate judgments. Finally, he needs feedback to inform him whether his changes are correct. The same kind of sequence is necessary for making behavioral changes, such as improving form in a sport, correcting faults in playing an instrument, or perfecting techniques of persuasion.

To illustrate the process of cognitive change, let us take as a rather gross example a person who is afraid of all strangers. When we explore his reactions, we may find that he is operating under the rule, "All strangers are unfriendly or hostile." In this case, the rule is wrong. On the other hand, he may realize that strangers vary, but he may not have learned to discriminate among friendly strangers, neutral strangers, and unfriendly strangers. In such a case, his trouble is in applying the rule, that is, in converting the available information in a given situation into an appropriate judgment.

It is obvious that not all people who think erroneously need or want to get their thinking straightened out. When a person's erroneous ideation disrupts his life or makes him feel miserable, then he becomes a candidate for some form of help.

The troubles or problems that stimulate a person to seek help may be manifested by distress of a subjective nature (such as anxiety or depression), a difficulty in his overt behavior (such as disabling inhibition or overaggressiveness), or a deficiency in his responses (for example, inability to experience or express warm feelings). The kinds of thinking that underlie these problems may be summarized as follows.

DIRECT, TANGIBLE DISTORTIONS OF REALITY

Distortions familiar to everybody are the thoughts of a paranoid patient who indiscriminately concludes when he sees other people (even people who are obviously friendly toward him): "Those people want to harm me." Or, as one patient once told me, "I killed President Kennedy."

Less obvious distortions of reality occur in all neuroses. For example, a depressed patient may say, "I have lost my ability to type, to read, to drive a car." However, when he becomes involved in the task, he may find his performance is still adequate. A depressed businessman complains that he is on the verge of bankruptcy, yet examination of his accounts indicates that he is completely solvent and, in fact, is prospering. The label "distortion of reality" is justified because an objective appraisal of the situation contradicts his appraisal.

Other examples of distortions that are relatively

simple to check are ideas such as, "I am getting fat" or "I am a burden to my family." Some judgments require greater work to authenticate; for example, "Nobody likes me." The therapeutic sessions, particularly when the patient has been trained to report his automatic thoughts, provide an excellent laboratory for exposing distortions. The therapist may readily identify certain distortions, for instance, when a patient toward whom he has warm feelings reports the thought that he believes the therapist dislikes him.

ILLOGICAL THINKING

The patient's appraisal of reality may not be distorted, but his system of making inferences or drawing conclusions from his observations is at fault: He hears distant noise and concludes someone has fired a gun at him. In such instances, the basic premises may be erroneous or the logical processes may be faulty. A depressed patient observed that a faucet was leaking in a bathroom, that the pilot light was out in the stove, and that one of the steps in the staircase was broken. He concluded, "The whole house is deteriorating." The house was in excellent condition (except for these minor problems); he had made a massive overgeneralization. In the same way, patients who have difficulties as a result of their overt behavior often start from inaccurate premises. Someone who consistently alienates potential friends because of his overaggressiveness may operate according to the rule, "If I don't push people around, they will push me around." A timid, inhibited person may be indiscriminately applying the principle, "If I open my mouth, everybody will jump on me."

THE THERAPEUTIC COLLABORATION

Certain factors are important in practically all forms of psychotherapy, but are crucial in cognitive therapy. An obvious primary component of effective psychotherapy is genuine collaboration between the therapist and patient. Moving blindly in separate directions, as sometimes happens, frustrates the therapist and distresses the patient. It is important to realize that the dispenser of the service (the therapist) and the recipient (the patient) may envision the therapeutic relationship quite differently. The patient, for instance, may visualize therapy as a molding of a lump of clay by an omnipotent and omniscient God figure. To minimize such hazards, the patient and therapist should reach a consensus regarding what problem requires help, the goal of therapy, and how they plan to reach that goal. Agreement regarding the nature and duration of therapy is important in determining the outcome. One study has shown, for instance, that a discrepancy between the patient's expectations and the kind of therapy he actually receives militates against a successful outcome. On the other hand, preliminary coaching of the patient about the type of therapy selected appeared to enhance its effectiveness (Orne and Wender, 1968).

Furthermore, the therapist needs to be tuned in to the vicissitudes of the patient's problems from session to session. Patients frequently formulate an "agenda" of topics they want to discuss at a particular session; if the therapist disregards this, he may impose an unnecessary strain on the relationship. For instance, a patient who is disturbed by a recent altercation with his wife may be alienated by the therapist's rigid adherence to a predetermined format such as desensitizing him to his subway phobia.

It is useful to conceive of the patient-therapist relationship as a joint effort. It is not the therapist's function to try to reform the patient; rather, his role is working with the patient against "*it,*" the patient's problem. Placing the emphasis on solving problems, rather than his presumed defects or bad habits, helps the patient to examine his difficulties with more detachment and makes him less prone to experience shame, a sense of inferiority, and defensiveness. The partnership concept helps the therapist to obtain valuable "feedback" about the efficacy of therapeutic techniques and further detailed information about the patient's thoughts and feelings. In employing systematic desensitization, for instance, I customarily ask for a detailed description of each image. The patient's report is often very informative and, on many occasions, reveals new problems that had not previously been identified. The partnership arrangement also reduces the patient's tendency to cast the therapist in the role of a superman. Investigators (Rogers, 1951; Truax, 1963) have found that if the therapist shows the following characteristics, a successful outcome is facilitated: genuine warmth, acceptance, and accurate empathy. By working with the patient as a collaborator, the therapist is more likely to show these characteristics than if he assumes a Godlike role.

ESTABLISHING CREDIBILITY

Problems often arise with regard to the suggestions and formulations offered by the therapist. Patients who view the therapist as a kind of superman are likely to accept his interpretations and suggestions as sacred pronouncements. Such bland ingestion of the therapist's hypotheses deprives the therapy of the corrective effect of critical evaluation by the patient.

A different type of problem is presented by patients who automatically react to the therapist's statements with suspicion or skepticism. Such a reaction is most pronounced in paranoid and severely depressed patients. In attempting to expose the distortions of reality, the therapist may become mired in the patient's deeply entrenched belief system. The therapist, therefore, must establish some common ground, find some point of agreement, and then attempt to extend the area of consensus from there. Depressed patients are often concerned that their emotional disorder will persist or get worse, and that they will not respond to therapy. If the therapist assumes a hearty optimistic attitude, the patient may decide that the therapist is either faking, doesn't really understand the gravity of the disorder, or is simply a fool. Similarly, trying to talk a paranoid patient out of his distorted views of reality may drive him to stronger belief in his paranoid ideas. Also, if the paranoid patient begins to regard the therapist as a member of the "opposition," he may assign the therapist a key role in his delusional system.

A more appropriate approach in establishing credibility is to convey a message such as: "You have certain ideas that upset you. They may or they may not be correct. Now let us examine some of them." By assuming a neutral stance, the therapist may then encourage the patient to express his distorted ideas and listen to them attentively. Later he sends up some "trial balloons" to determine whether the patient is ready to examine the evidence regarding these distortions.

One of the reasons that persecutory ideas of paranoids and fixed self-debasement ideas of depressives have been regarded traditionally as impermeable to psychotherapy is that the therapist has attempted to correct the patient's thinking prematurely. Even fixed delusions, however, may eventually become amenable to modification if the therapist is sensitive and patient (Beck, 1952; Davison, 1966; Salzman, 1960; Schwartz, 1963).

Studies by social psychologists indicate that dogmatism tends to widen the gap between persons with different opinions, and to make them more extreme and rigid in their opposing views. A similar phenomenon occurs in psychotherapy. Because of the patient's reluctance openly to express his disagreement, a dogmatic therapist may be deceived into assuming they have reached a consensus. Even the careful therapist, however, needs to be vigilant to any cues indicative of the patient's disagreement. A method for determining whether the patient indeed does agree with statements by the therapist is illustrated in the following interchange:

Therapist: Now that you've heard my formulation of the problem, what do you think of it?

Patient: It sounds O.K. to me.

Therapist: While I was talking, did you have any feeling that there might be some parts that you disagree with?

Patient: I'm not sure.

Therapist: You would tell me if you were uncertain about some of the things I said, wouldn't you?...You know, some patients are reluctant to disagree with their doctor.

Patient: Well, I could see that what you said was logical, but I'm not really sure I believe it.

Statements such as this usually suggest that the patient disagrees, at least in part, with the therapist. The therapist should proceed to ascertain the patient's reservations and encourage him to rebut the therapist's formulation.

Many patients appear to agree with the therapist because of their fears of challenging him and their need to please him. A clue to such superficial consensus is provided by the patient who says, "I agree with you intellectually but not emotionally." Such a statement generally indicates that the therapist's comments or interpretations may seem logical to the patient, but that they do not penetrate the patient's basic belief system (Ellis, 1962). The patient continues to operate according to his faulty ideas. Moreover, strongly authoritative remarks that appeal to the patient's yearning for explanations for his misery may set the stage for disillusionment when the patient finds loopholes in the therapist's formulations. The therapist's confidence in his role as an expert requires a strong admixture of humility. Psychotherapy often involves a good deal of trial-and-error, experimenting with several approaches or formulations to determine which fit the best.

Delusional thinking obviously tests the confidence of a patient in the therapist. It is generally wise not to try to attack a delusion directly. Even if the therapist does not challenge it, he can help the patient cope with it. For example, an elderly man who had a serious physical illness developed the delusion that his elderly wife was carrying on an affair with his young physician. The patient therefore started to berate his wife and accuse her of infidelity. His accusations were so disturbing to his wife that she seriously considered leaving him. The patient's psychiatrist said to him: "I have no evidence regarding the accuracy of your accusations about your wife, but you should consider the consequences of your behavior. What will happen to you if you continue to accuse her and berate her?" The patient initially replied that he didn't care. The psychiatrist then said, "If she leaves you, who will take care of you?" This question forced the patient to consider the possible consequences of his actions. He stopped making accusations and his relationship with his wife improved. In fact, the patient felt more friendly toward his wife. It is also possible that by his stopping his accusations, the delusion of infidelity may have become attenuated—although there is no direct evidence to support this conjecture.

In less extreme cases, it is possible to deal more directly with the irrational ideas. However, the therapist must assess the "latitude of acceptance" of the patient for statements challenging his distorted concepts. Being told that his ideas are wrong might antagonize the patient; but, he might respond favorably to a question such as "Is there another way of interpreting your wife's behavior?" As long as the therapist's attempts at clarification are within an acceptable range, the problem of a credibility gap is minimized.

PROBLEM REDUCTION

Many patients come to the therapist with a host of symptoms or problems. To solve each one of the problems in isolation from the others might very well take a lifetime. A patient may seek help for a variety of ailments such as headaches, insomnia, and anxiety, in addition to interpersonal problems. Identifying problems with similar causes and grouping them together is termed "problem reduction." Once the multifarious difficulties are condensed, the therapist can select the appropriate techniques for each group of problems.

Let us take as an example the patient with multiple phobias. A woman described in Chapter 7 was greatly handicapped by a fear of elevators, tunnels, hills, closed spaces, riding in an open car, riding in an airplane, swimming, walking fast or running, strong winds, and hot, muggy days. Treating each phobia separately with the technique of systematic desensitization might have required innumerable therapeutic sessions. However, it was possible to find a common denominator for her symptoms: an overriding fear of suffocation. She believed that each of the phobic situations presented substantial risk of deprivation of air and consequent suffocation. The therapy was focused directly on this central fear.

The principle of problem reduction is also applicable to a constellation of symptoms that comprise a specific disorder such as depression. By concentrating on certain key components of the disorder, such as low self-esteem or negative expectations, the therapy can produce improvement in mood, overt behavior, appetite, and sleeping pattern. One patient, for instance, revealed that whenever he was in a gratifying situation, he would get some kind of "kill-joy" thought: When he began to feel pleasure from listening to music, he would think, "This record will be over soon," and his pleasure would disappear. When he discovered that he was enjoying a movie, a date with a girl, or just walking, he would think:

"This will end soon," and immediately his satisfaction was squelched. In this case, a thought pattern that he could not enjoy things because they would end became the focus of the therapy.

In another case the main focus was the patient's overabsorption in the negative aspects of her life and her selective inattention to positive occurrences. The therapy consisted of having her write down and report back positive experiences. She was surprised to find how many positive, gratifying experiences she had had and subsequently forgotten about.

Another form of problem reduction is the identification of the first link in a chain of symptoms. An interesting feature is that the first link may be a relatively small and easily eradicable problem that leads to consequences that are disabling. For analogy, a person may writhe with pain and be unable to walk, eat, talk at length, or perform minimal constructive activities—because of a speck in the eye. The "speck in the eye" syndrome probably occurs more frequently among psychiatric patients than is generally realized. Because of delay in identifying and dealing with the initial problem, however, the ensuing difficulties become deeply entrenched. A mother who was afraid to leave her children at home with a babysitter continued to be housebound long after the children reached maturity.

By a painstaking review of the patient's symptoms and past history it is often possible to delineate the causal sequences. It is generally most parsimonious to concentrate on those factors found to be primary, that is, that are causative in producing the other symptoms. A graduate student with a long-standing history of depression, for instance, had received psychotherapy consisting of fruitless attempts by the therapist to increase his self-esteem and to neutralize his self-criticisms. In addition, he received trials of practically every antidepressant medication on the market. Nonetheless, the patient continued to feel sad and lonely, was preoccupied with self-derogatory thoughts, had sleep disturbance, loss of appetite, and a chronic state of fatigue.

After detailed analysis of the patient's past and present circumstances, the following pattern emerged. This young man had had a number of long-standing phobias: fears of going out alone, of open spaces, of social rejection. He had compensated for these during his school years by virtue of the fact that, since he was living at home, he had always been able to find someone to accompany him to school. Also, his friends had helped to buffer his fear of rejection by joining him in new social situations. Through this system of compensations and buffers, he had been able to go through college and have a satisfying social life. By circumventing his fears, he had not been disabled by his phobias.

His depression became manifest after he moved to a distant city to attend graduate school. Left on his own, he began to experience intense anxiety. When he would start to walk to class, he feared he would experience a physical catastrophe and that there would be nobody there to help him. He felt safer in his apartment where he was always close to a telephone and could call several physicians with whom he had made contact. Although he managed to force himself to go to his classes, traveling was accompanied by considerable anxiety, and he could barely wait to return to his room when classes were over. He did not make new friends because his anxiety was stirred up whenever he attempted to form a relationship with another student. As a result, he avoided anxiety-producing situations as much as possible. The cumulative effect of the complete deprivation of social interaction was feelings of loneliness, pessimism, apathy, and physiological signs of depression.

On the basis of this reconstruction of the causal sequence, we concentrated primarily on the phobias rather than on the depression *per se.* Techniques used to help him overcome his phobias consisted of systematic desensitization in which he imaged scenes of physical catastrophe and also a separate set of scenes of social rejection. He was encouraged to resist his avoidance tendencies, and he exposed himself increasingly to the situations that frightened him. Eventually he was able to leave his apartment without anxiety and to engage in conversation with a stranger. Although his symptoms of depression were somewhat alleviated by his sense of accomplishment, they were still present in significant amounts. As he overcame his phobic reactions, however, he was gradually able to establish new relationships and to obtain the gratification he missed. As his satisfactions from social activity increased, his depression disappeared.

LEARNING TO LEARN

As pointed out in the previous section, it is not necessary for a psychotherapist to help a patient solve every problem that troubles him. Nor is it necessary to anticipate all the problems that may occur after the termination of therapy and to try to work them out in advance. The kind of therapeutic collaboration previously described is conducive to the patient's developing new ways to learn from his experiences and to solve problems. In a sense the patient is "learning to learn." This process has been labeled deutero-learning (Bateson, 1942).

The problem-solving approach to psychotherapy removes much of the responsibility from the therapist and engages the patient more actively in working on his difficulties. By reducing the patient's dependency on the therapist, this approach increases the patient's self-confidence and self-esteem. More important, perhaps, is the fact that the patient's active participation in defining the problem and considering various options yields more ample information than would otherwise be available. His participation in making the decision helps him implement it.

I have explained the problem-solving concept to patients in somewhat the following way: "One of the goals of therapy is to help you learn new ways of approaching problems. Then, as problems come up, you can apply the formulas that you have already learned. For instance, in learning arithmetic you simply learned the fundamental rules. It was not necessary to learn every single possible addition and subtraction. Once you had learned the operations, you could apply them to any arithmetic problem."

To illustrate "learning to learn," let us consider the practical and interpersonal problems that contribute to a patient's various symptoms. A woman, for instance, discovered she was constantly plagued with headaches, feelings of tension, abdominal pain, and insomnia. By focusing on her problems at work and at home, the patient was able to find some solutions for them and became less prone to experience symptoms. As was hoped, she was able to generalize these practical lessons to solving other problems of living, so that it was not necessary for us to work on all her problems in therapy.

Among the types of problems that had caused the symptoms were the following. She always felt tense when she was at work because her supervisor was hypercritical. Although the patient's performance was at a high level, she was always afraid of making a mistake because of the wrath that it might evoke from the supervisor. The patient could not, on her own, devise a way out of this situation. We rehearsed a number of approaches she might use in discussing the problem directly with her supervisor. When she felt ready, she told her supervisor: "I am always tense when you are around because I'm afraid you're going to jump on me. When you jump on me it only makes my performance worse. I was hoping I could talk to you about this." The supervisor was surprised to hear this, and subsequently was less critical of the patient.

The patient also learned from this experience that she could stand up to other people, and in other analogous situations was able to deal with her fear of criticism by being more assertive. In addition, her increasing self-esteem made her less sensitive to criticism.

"Learning to learn" consists of much more than the patient's adopting a few techniques that can be used in a wide variety of situations. Basically, this approach attempts to remove obstacles that have prevented the patient from profiting from experience and from developing adequate ways of dealing with their internal and external problems. Most of the patients have been blocked in their psychosocial development by certain maladaptive attitudes and patterns of behavior. For instance, the woman with the numerous problems at work and at home had a characteristic response when she was confronted with sensitive interpersonal relations or new practical problems: "I don't know what to do." As a result of therapy, each successful experience tended to erode this negative attitude. Consequently, she was enabled to draw on her ingenuity in meeting and mastering completely different situations.

Patients generally try to avoid situations that cause them uneasiness. Consequently, they do not develop the trial-and-error techniques that are prerequisite to solving many problems. Or by staying out of difficult situations, they do not learn how to rid themselves of their tendency to distort or exaggerate. A person who stays close to home because he fears strangers does not learn how to test the validity of his fears or to discriminate between "safe" strangers and "dangerous" strangers. Through therapy he can learn to "reality-test" not only these fears but other fears as well.

The sense of mastery from solving one problem frequently inspires the patient to approach and solve other problems that he has long avoided. Thus, a bonus of successful therapy is not only freedom from the original problems, but a thorough psychological change that prepares him to meet new challenges.

CHAPTER 10

Techniques of Cognitive Therapy

> *The problem of freedom in the psychological rather than the political sense of the word is in large measure a technical problem. It is not enough to wish to become the master, it is not even enough to work hard at achieving such mastery. Correct knowledge as to the best means of achieving mastery is also essential.*— Aldous Huxley

EXPERIMENTAL METHOD

The process of helping a patient identify and correct his distortions requires the application of certain principles of epistemology: the nature, limits, and criteria of knowledge. The therapist, directly or indirectly, conveys certain principles to the patient. First, a perception of reality is not the same as reality itself; at best, it is a rough approximation of reality. The patient's sampling of reality is restricted by the inherent limitations of his sensory functions—seeing, hearing, smelling, etc. Second, his interpretations of his sensory input are dependent on inherently fallible cognitive processes such as integrating and differentiating the stimuli. Physiological and psychological processes can substantially alter perception and comprehension of reality.

As is well known, distortion may occur when a person is under the influence of drugs, in a state of fatigue or diminished consciousness, or in a state of high arousal. We have also seen that appraisal of reality can be flawed by unrealistic patterns of thought. In anxiety neurosis, for instance, even innocuous stimuli are integrated in such a way as to suggest danger. A prerequisite for applying psychological techniques to alleviate this neurosis is the patient's ability to accept the distinctions between external reality (the innocuous stimuli) and the psychological phenomenon (the appraisal of danger). Intoxicated patients and acutely psychotic (delusional) patients are generally not able to accept or make this distinction.

In addition, the patient needs to be capable of testing hypotheses before accepting them as valid. Reliable knowledge depends ultimately on having sufficient information so that a choice can be made among alternative hypotheses. A housewife hears a door slam: Several hypotheses occur to her: "It may be Sally returning from school." "It might be a burglar." "It might be the wind that blew the door shut." The favored hypothesis should depend on her taking into account all the relevant circumstances. The logical process of hypothesis testing may be disrupted, however, by the housewife's psychological set. If her thinking is dominated by the concept of danger, she might jump to the conclusion, "It is a burglar." She makes an arbitrary inference. Although such an inference is not necessarily incorrect, it is based primarily on internal cognitive processes rather than actual information. If she then runs and hides, she postpones or forfeits the opportunity to disprove (or confirm) the hypothesis.

RECOGNIZING MALADAPTIVE IDEATION

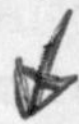

As pointed out in previous chapters, emotional reactions, motivations, and overt behavior are guided by thinking. A person may not be fully aware of the automatic thoughts that influence to a large extent how he acts, what he feels, and how much he enjoys his experiences. With some training, however, he may increase his awareness of these thoughts and learn to pinpoint them with a high degree of regularity. It is possible to perceive a thought, focus on it, and evaluate it just as one can identify and reflect on a sensation (such as pain) or an external stimulus (such as a verbal statement).

The term "maladaptive thoughts" is applied to ideation that interferes with the ability to cope with life experiences, unnecessarily disrupts internal harmony, and produces inappropriate or excessive emotional reactions that are painful. In cognitive therapy, the patient focuses on those thoughts or images that produce unnecessary discomfort or suffering or lead to self-defeating behavior. In applying the term "maladaptive," it is important that the therapist be wary of imposing his own value system on the patient. The term is generally applicable if both the patient and the therapist are able to agree that these automatic thoughts interfere with the patient's well-being or with the attainment of his important objectives.

Possible exceptions to this definition immediately spring to mind. Is a disturbing thought considered maladaptive if it is consonant with reality? It would seem difficult to justify applying the label "maladaptive" to an accurate appraisal of danger (and its associated anxiety) or to the recognition of a real loss and the resulting arousal of grief. Yet, under some circumstances, even such reality-oriented ideation may be regarded as maladaptive because of its interference with functioning. For example, steeplejacks, bridge-workers and mountain climbers may not only suffer serious discomfort, but may be subjected to greatly increased risk by a stream of thoughts or images about falling. Such ideation not only distracts them from concentrating on their task, but the associated anxiety may lead to swaying, dizziness, and trembling that may disturb their balance. Similarly, a surgeon distracted by thoughts of making a slip with his scalpel may endanger his patient's life. People engaged in hazardous activities generally acquire the ability to disregard or extinguish such thoughts. With experience, they seem to form a psychological buffer that diminishes the force and frequency of the thoughts. The presence of this buffer separates the seasoned veteran from the novice.

In actual clinical practice, the therapist is rarely forced to make a fine distinction between maladaptive and realistic thoughts. The distortions or self-defeating characteristics are usually obvious enough to justify calling them maladaptive. A man, depressed for years after the death of his wife, went beyond the realistic consequences of the loss and was preoccupied with extreme ideas such as, "It's my fault that she died," or "I can't exist without her," or "I will never find any satisfaction." Similarly, a student with pre-examination jitters thought, "It will be the end for me if I fail; I will never be able to face my friends," or "I will end up on skid row." After the examination, he easily realized the exaggerated, unrealistic nature of these thoughts.

Ellis (1962) refers to this kind of maladaptive thinking as "internalized statements" or "self-statements" and he describes them to the patient as "things you tell yourself." Maultsby (1968) uses the term "self-talk" to label these thoughts. Such explanations are of practical value in that they imply to the patient that the maladaptive thoughts are voluntary, and therefore he can voluntarily switch them off or change them. While recognizing the practical usefulness of this terminology, I prefer the term "automatic thoughts," because it more accurately reflects the way the thoughts are experienced. The person perceives these thoughts as though they arise by reflex—without any prior reflection or reasoning; and they impress him as plausible and valid. They can be compared to statements made to a believing child by his parent. The patient can frequently be trained to terminate this kind of thinking, but in severe cases, especially psychoses, physiological interventions such as administration of drugs or electroconvulsive therapy may be required to stop the maladaptive thoughts.

The force and prominence of maladaptive thoughts appear to increase in measure with the severity of the patient's disturbance. In severe disorders, the thoughts are generally salient and may, in fact, occupy the center of the ideational field. This phenomenon may be observed in acute or severe cases of depression, anxiety, or paranoid states. In depression, the patient may have no voluntary control over ruminations such as "I'm no good. . . My insides are gone. . . Everything bad happens to me." Analogous types of preoccupations with danger occur in anxiety states and preoccupation with abuse in paranoid states.

On the other hand, obsessional patients who are not acutely or severely disturbed may be very conscious of certain types of repetitive statements. These incessant thoughts are diagnostic indications of this disorder. Moreover, people who are free of neurosis may experience similar preoccupations. A mother alarmed about her sick child or a student concerned about an imminent examination is apt to experience the relentless repetition of unpleasant thoughts about the particular problem. Any person who has such "worries" can attest to how involuntary they seem.

A person experiencing a mild disturbance in his feelings or behavior may not be aware of the automatic thoughts—even though they are accessible to consciousness. In such cases, the automatic thoughts do not attract his attention—although they can exert an influence on how he feels and acts. By concentrating on the thoughts, however, he can easily recognize them. We can observe this phenomenon in people who have recovered from the acute phase of a psychological disturbance or who are only mildly disturbed.

People who characteristically avoid situations that upset them, such as phobics, will not be conscious of their maladaptive ideation as long as they maintain a comfortable distance from the threatening situations. However, when they are forced into the situation or imagine themselves in the situation, these maladaptive thoughts become activated, and can readily be identified.

When a patient states he had never been aware of his

automatic thoughts until after he had been trained to observe them, we are faced with a philosophical problem: How can a person be unaware of something in his field of consciousness? Yet, many of us have had the experience of having been exposed to a particular stimulus but having no conscious awareness of it until it was pointed out to us. At that point, we might remark, "I realize that it was there all the time, but I just did not notice it before." In such situations, it seems that the perception occurred but we did not pay any attention to it. Yet, this perception may have influenced our train of thought or feelings. A person having difficulty in falling asleep may not be aware that his restlessness is influenced by noxious sounds such as the loud ticking of a clock or heavy traffic. Similarly, automatic thoughts occur within the realm of consciousness, but, until he has been trained, the person may not observe them. By shifting his attention to these thoughts he becomes more aware of them and can specify their content.

FILLING IN THE BLANK

When the automatic thoughts are in the center of awareness, there is no problem in identifying them. In cases of mild to moderate neurosis, a program of instructions and practice sessions is generally necessary to train the patient to delineate those thoughts. Sometimes, by fantasizing the traumatic situation, the individual may stir up such thoughts.

A basic procedure for helping a patient identify his automatic thoughts is to train him to observe the sequence of external events and his reactions to them. The patient may report a number of circumstances in which he felt unaccountably upset. Usually, there is a gap between the stimulus and emotional response. The emotional upset becomes understandable if he can recollect the thoughts that occurred during this gap.

Ellis describes the following techniques for explaining this procedure to the patient. He calls the sequence: "A, B, C." "A" is the "Activating stimulus" and "C" is the excessive, inappropriate "Conditioned response." "B" is the Blank in the patient's mind, which, when he fills it in, serves as a bridge between "A" and "C." Filling in the blank, which derives from the patient's belief system, becomes the therapeutic task.

One patient outlined the sequence of A, seeing an old friend, and C, experiencing sadness. Another patient reported the sequence: A, he heard a report about somebody being killed in an automobile accident, and C, felt anxiety. In these instances the patients were able to replay the events in slow motion, as it were, and could then successfully recall the thoughts that had occurred in the gap. Seeing the old friend had elicited *B,* the following sequence of thoughts: "If I greet Bob, he may not remember me...He may snub me...It's been so long, we won't have anything in common. It won't be like old times." These thoughts evoked the sad feelings. The patient who felt anxious after witnessing the auto accident was able to fill in the blank when he recalled having had a fantasy image of himself as the victim.

The A B C sequence may be illustrated by the common fear of dogs. A person may assert that although he has no reason for fearing dogs, he experiences anxiety whenever he is exposed to them. One such patient was puzzled by the fact that he became frightened when near a dog even when there was no possibility of his being attacked. He would feel nervous when a dog was chained or fenced in, or when a dog was obviously too small to injure him. I recommended that he focus on whatever thoughts occurred to him the next time he saw a dog—any dog.

At the next interview, the patient reported having seen a number of dogs between appointments. He reported a phenomenon that he had not noticed previously—mainly, that each time he saw a dog he had a thought such as, "It's going to bite me." By focusing on the intervening thoughts, he was able to understand why he felt anxious: He automatically regarded every dog as dangerous. He commented that he experienced the fear of being bitten even when he saw a miniature poodle. He stated, "I realized how ridiculous it was to think that a small poodle could hurt me." He also recognized that when he saw a large dog on a leash he would think of the most deleterious eventualities: "The dog will jump up and bite out one of my eyes." "It will jump up and bite my neck and kill me." Within three weeks, the patient was able to overcome his long-standing fear by repeatedly recognizing his thoughts when exposed to dogs.

The technique of "filling in the blank" can be of great help to patients disturbed by excessive shame, anxiety, anger, or sadness in interpersonal situations, or handicapped by fears of specific locations or structures. A college student avoided public gatherings because of inexplicable feelings of shame, anxiety, and sadness in these situations. After having been trained to recognize and record his cognitions, he reported having had these thoughts in social situations: "Nobody will want to talk to me... They think I look pathetic... I'm just a misfit." After having these thoughts, he experienced feelings of humiliation, anxiety, and sadness and would have a strong desire to leave.

Another patient complained that he became almost uncontrollably angry whenever he had interchanges with strangers—when making purchases, asking for information, or just conversing. After two training sessions, he reported that he recognized intermediate thoughts such as, "He's pushing me around," "He thinks I'm a pushover," "She's trying to take advantage of me." Immediately after experiencing these thoughts, he would feel angry at the person toward whom they were directed. Until this time, he had not realized that he had a tendency to regard other people as adversaries. Another patient felt chronically irritated in the presence of other people without realizing why. After focusing on his thoughts, he realized he was having continuous critical ideas about these people.

Many times, maladaptive ideation occurs in a pictorial form instead of, or in addition to, the verbal form (Beck, 1970c): A woman with a fear of walking alone had images of having a heart attack and being left helpless and dying on the street. Then she would feel acute anxiety. Another woman who experienced a surge of anxiety when driving across a bridge recognized that the anxiety was preceded by a pictorial image of her car breaking through the guard rail and her falling off the bridge. A student discovered that his anxiety at leaving his dormitory at night was triggered by visual fantasies of being attacked by gangsters.

DISTANCING AND DECENTERING

Some patients who have learned to identify their automatic thoughts recognize their unreliable and maladaptive nature spontaneously. With successive observations of their thoughts, they became increasingly able to view these thoughts objectively. The process of regarding thoughts objectively is labeled *distancing*. The concept of distancing is derived from its usage to denote the ability of patients who are administered a projective test, such as Rorschach's ink-blot test, to maintain the distinction between the ink-blot configurations and the association or fantasy stimulated by the figure. Patients who are "carried away" by strong emotional reactions to the perceptions aroused by the configuration are often found to regard the ink blot as though it were the same as the object or scenes it conjured up. The patient who is able to withdraw his attention from this association and to perceive this stimulus as simply an ink blot is said to be able to "take distance" from the blot.

In an analogous way, a person who can examine his automatic thoughts as psychological phenomena rather than as identical to reality is exercising the capacity for distancing. Take, for example, a patient who, for no justifiable reason, has the thought, "That man is my enemy." If he automatically equates the thought with reality, his distancing is poor. If he can regard the idea as a hypothesis or inference, rather than accept it as fact, he is distancing well.

Concepts such as distancing, reality testing, authenticating observations, and validating conclusions, are related to epistemology. Distancing involves being able to make the distinction between "I believe" (an opinion that is subject to validation) and "I know" (an "irrefutable" fact). The ability to make this distinction is of critical importance in modifying those sectors of the patient's reactions that are subject to distortion.

In various psychological disorders—anxiety, depression, paranoid states—major distortion in thinking results from the patient's proclivity to personalize events that have no causal connection to him. A depressed man blames himself for the fact that a family picnic he had scheduled had to be cancelled because of rain. An anxious woman sees a burned building and thinks that *her* house may be on fire. A paranoid patient sees a frown on the face of a passerby and concludes that person wants to harm him. The technique of prying the patient loose from his pattern of regarding himself as the focal point of all events is called decentering. The successful application of this method is illustrated in the following case (Schuyler, 1973).

A graduate student had a good deal of anxiety prior to taking examinations. His anxiety was exacerbated because he interpreted the physiological symptoms (shortness of breath, tachycardia, etc.) as signs of an impending heart attack. According to his philosophy of predestination, he decided that fate had singled him out for a special hardship. He passed the written examination for an advanced degree but failed the oral examination. Although he realized that his anxiety had interfered with his oral examination, he interpreted the failure itself as evidence that fate was against him.

At the time he was to take his oral examination a second time, there was considerable snow on the ground. On the way to the examination, he slipped and fell. He then became quite anxious. He was able to identify the relevant thought: "The snow has been put there so that I would fall." Then he recalled what his therapist had told him about his tendency to personalize external events. He looked around and saw that other people were slipping, that automobiles were skidding on the ice, and that even a dog had slid and fallen. As he was struck by the realization that the snow was not a special hardship directed at him, his anxiety disappeared.

AUTHENTICATING CONCLUSIONS

It generally does not occur to a person to question the validity of his thoughts. He tends to regard ideas as though they were a microcosm of the outside world. He attaches the same truth value to his thought as he does to his perception of the external world.

Even after a patient is able to make a clear distinction between his internal mental processes and the outside world that stimulates them, it is still necessary to educate him regarding the procedures for acquiring accurate knowledge. People continually set up hypotheses and draw inferences. They tend to equate an inference with reality and to accept a hypothesis as though it were a fact. Under ordinary circumstances, they might be able to function adequately because their ideation may be sufficiently in phase with the real world so as not to substantially interfere with their adjustment.

In cases of neurosis, the distorted concepts can have a disabling effect. These distorted concepts lead to faulty thinking in certain circumscribed areas of experience. In these particular sectors they tend to make global undifferentiated judgments instead of the fine discriminations that are necessary to keep in tune with reality. As indicated in Chapter 4, the patient frequently detours logic and leaps to arbitrary inferences, overgeneralizations, and magnifications.

The psychotherapist can apply certain techniques to determine whether the patients' conclusions are inaccurate or unjustified. Since the patient has been habitually making distortions, the therapeutic procedure consists essentially of exploring his conclusions and testing them against reality. The therapist works with the patient to apply the rules of evidence to his conclusions. This consists initially of checking his observations and then following the route to the conclusions.

CHANGING THE RULES

We have seen that people apply rules (formulas, equations, premises) in regulating their own lives and in trying to modify the behavior of other people. Moreover, they label, interpret, and evaluate according to sets of rules. When these rules are framed in absolute terms, are unrealistic, or are used inappropriately or excessively, they frequently produce maladjustment. The ultimate result is often some kind disturbance: anxiety, depression, phobia, mania, paranoid state, obsession. When the rules lead to difficulties, they are by definition maladaptive.

Ellis (1962) refers to such rules as "irrational ideas." His term, while powerful, is not accurate. The ideas are generally not irrational but are too absolute, broad, and extreme; too highly personalized; and are used too arbitrarily to help the patient to handle the exigencies of his life. To be of greater use, the rules need to be remolded so that they are more precise and accurate, less egocentric, and more elastic. When rules are discovered to be false, self-defeating, or unworkable, they have to be dropped from the repertoire. In such cases, the therapist and patient work together to substitute more realistic and adaptive rules.

Inasmuch as other writers have used terms such as

attitudes, ideas, concepts and constructs to refer to what we have called rules, those terms will be used interchangeably in the following discussion. Irrespective of terminology used, many therapists have reported that helping the patient to modify his maladaptive ideas or to substitute more realistic attitudes has led to the disappearance of crippling anxieties, phobias, and depressions. Therapists sometimes overlook the obvious truth that if a patient's incorrect assumptions or personal mythology are not related to his difficulties, it is not necessary to change them. The therapist's mandate does not require that he educate his patient to be a Renaissance man.

The content of the rules for coding experiences and steering behavior seem to revolve around two main axes: *danger versus safety* and *pain versus pleasure*. Patients' difficulties arise in their assessments of risk and safety or in their conceptions of pain and gratification.

The rules dealing with safety and danger include physical harm and psychological harm (see Chapter 7). The concerns about physical harm cover a broad range of "dangerous situations": being assaulted or killed by other people or animals; being injured or killed by falling from high places, or by collisions (as in automobile accidents); suffocating or starving by being deprived of air or food; or being afflicted by a wide host of diseases and poisons. It is obvious that these noxious events occur in the real world. For purposes of survival, people use their mental rule books to interpret dangerous situations and to assess the degree of risk. The person who encounters difficulties either by being unnecessarily apprehensive or by behaving recklessly does not have the correct rules, or else does not apply them correctly.

Psychosocial harm covers the varieties of hurt

feelings, humiliations, embarrassments, and sadness that occur after a person has been insulted, criticized, or rejected. It should be noted that these feelings can occur when a person simply *thinks* he has been insulted, criticized or rejected—when indeed he has not been. Furthermore, unlike physical injury, which generally provides some reliable index of the degree of trauma (for example, bleeding, specific localized pain), rejection or criticism do not leave any telltale marks. The person simply feels bad but we cannot discern from this reaction whether the bad feeling is based on a real or on a fancied insult.

In order to minimize danger, people generally apply rules to estimate the probabilities and degree of harm and the likelihood of dealing successfully with the threat. The ratio between the potential harm and coping mechanisms may be labeled the risk. If a person overestimates the risk, he is unnecessarily anxious and may lead a constricted life. If he underestimates the risk, he is more prone to having accidents.

The complexities of interpersonal relations and the lack of a reliable index of another person's intentions to cause hurt add a fuzziness to the rules used in interpersonal situations. Some people regard themselves as highly vulnerable in all interpersonal contacts and thus feel constantly on the razor's edge. Conversely, those who are oblivious to signals from other people, of course, may regularly get into interpersonal difficulties.

Because most problems presented by patients seem to arise in the context of interpersonal relations, some of the common interpersonal attitudes will be considered first. Interpersonal dangers are epitomized by a rule such as the following: "It would be awful for someone to form a low opinion of me." The other person might be a close friend, a parent, a peer, remote acquaintance, or a stranger. In clinical practice, we find that our patients are generally most afraid of being devalued by members of their peer group—their classmates, fellow workers, colleagues, or friends. Many patients, however, are even more afraid of the prospect of appearing ridiculous to strangers. They are apprehensive of the reactions of clerks in stores, waiters, taxi drivers, passengers on a bus, or passersby on a street. It is possible that the strangers' reactions are more threatening because these patients have not learned from direct experience what to expect.

A person may dread a situation in which he considers himself vulnerable to other people's adverse criticisms of him (either overt or unexpressed). He is sensitized to situations in which some "weakness" or "fault" of his might be exposed. He might be afraid of disapproval for not expressing himself well, behaving too aggressively, appearing different from other people—or even seeming to be afraid of disapproval. In more extreme cases, he may be afraid of losing control: being too emotional, fainting, or acting insane.

All kinds of negative reactions may be envisioned, ranging from stony stares to denunciations. It is essential to understand that the person regards such reactions from other people as very bad. When patients are asked why it might be so bad to be criticized by a stranger, it becomes apparent that they simply regard this as bad *by definition.* They are usually at a loss to explain why it is so bad. They have a vague notion that a rejection or criticism will in some way permanently and irreversibly damage their social image and self-image.

A therapeutic approach to dealing with such fears of criticism is illustrated by the case of a medical student who was inhibited in numerous situations in which self-assertion was necessary, for example, asking a stranger for directions, checking a cashier's tally of his bill, refusing to do something asked of him, asking somebody to do him a favor, or speaking in front of a group. The following interview excerpts illustrate the approach used to help the student:

> *Patient:* I have to give a talk before my class tomorrow and I'm scared stiff.
> *Therapist:* What are you afraid of?
> *Patient:* I think I'll make a fool of myself.
> *Therapist:* Suppose you do. . . make a fool of yourself. . . Why is that so bad?
> *Patient:* I'll never live it down.
> *Therapist:* "Never" is a long time. . . Now look here, suppose they ridicule you. Can you die from it?
> *Patient:* Of course not.
> *Therapist:* Suppose they decide you're the worst public speaker that ever lived. . . Will this ruin your future career?
> *Patient:* No. . . But it would be nice if I could be a good speaker.
> *Therapist:* Sure it would be nice. But if you flubbed it, would your parents or your wife disown you?
> *Patient:* No. . . They're very sympathetic.
> *Therapist:* Well, what would be so awful about it?
> *Patient:* I would feel pretty bad.
> *Therapist:* For how long?
> *Patient:* For about a day or two.
> *Therapist:* And then what?
> *Patient:* Then I'd be O.K.
> *Therapist:* So you're scaring yourself just as though your fate hangs in the balance.

Patient: That's right. It does feel as though my whole future is at stake.

Therapist: Now somewhere along the line, your thinking got fouled up...and you tend to regard any failure as though it's the end of the world... What you have to do is get your failures labeled correctly—as failure to reach a goal, not as disaster. You have to start to challenge your wrong premises.

In the next appointment, after the patient had given his talk—which, as he predicted, was somewhat disorganized because of his fears—we reviewed his notions about his failure.

Therapist: How do you feel now?

Patient: I feel better...but I was down in the dumps for a few days.

Therapist: What do you think now about your notion that giving a fumbling talk is a catastrophe?

Patient: Of course, it isn't a catastrophe.

Therapist: What is it then?

Patient: It's unpleasant, but I will survive.

The patient was coached in changing his notion that a failure is a catastrophe. He found that he had much less anticipatory anxiety prior to his next talk a week later, and felt more comfortable during the talk. At the next session, he completely agreed that he had attached too much importance to what the reactions of his classmates might be. The following interchange occurred:

Patient: I felt much better during my last speech... I guess it's a matter of experience.

Therapist: Did you get some glimmer of the notion

that it really isn't vital for the most part what people think of you?

Patient: If I'm going to be a doctor, I've got to make a good impression on my patients.

Therapist: Whether you're a good doctor depends on how well you diagnose and treat your patients, not how good you are at public speaking.

Patient: Well, I know I'm good with patients—and I guess that's what counts.

The rest of the therapy was devoted to challenging his maladaptive attitudes that produced discomfort in other situations. The patient articulated the new attitude he was acquiring when he said: "I really can see now how ridiculous it is to be concerned about perfect strangers. I will never see them again. So what difference does it make what they will think of me?"

Assumptions relevant to physical fears may be challenged and modified in a similar way. Often the maladaptive attitude becomes activated only as the patient approaches the feared situation, but the attitude may also be mobilized by having the patient discuss the phobic situation or imagine himself in the situation. (The imagining of the situation is one of the basic techniques of Wolpe's systematic desensitization.) The underlying rule is framed somewhat like this: "If I climb the stairs (drive through a tunnel, go into a crowded store, go to the top of a tall building), I will have a heart attack (will suffocate, will faint, will fall out)."

Since many patients do not attach much credence to the danger when they are in the safety of the therapist's office, it is useful to employ a strategy that will activate the fear and then help the patient to deal with the attitude. In Chapter 7 we noted that a man who feared air travel believed the chance of a crash to be minimal until he began to plan a trip. In the following instance, a woman was troubled by fear of being in crowded places:

> *Therapist:* What are you afraid of when you're in a crowded place?
> *Patient:* I'm afraid I won't be able to catch my breath...
> *Therapist:* And?
> *Patient:* ...I'll pass out.
> *Therapist:* Just pass out?
> *Patient:* All right, I know it sounds silly but I'm afraid I will just stop breathing...and die.
> *Therapist:* Right now, what do you think are the probabilities that you will suffocate and die?
> *Patient:* Right now, it seems like one chance in a thousand.

The patient was then instructed in the following technique. She was told to make notations on a pad of the probabilities of dying as she approached the crowded store. At the next interview, the patient brought in the following notations:

1. Leaving my house—chances of dying in store—1 in 1,000
2. Driving into town—chances of dying in store—1 in 100
3. Parking car in lot—chances of dying in store—1 in 50
4. Walking to store—chances of dying in store—1 in 10
5. Entering store—chances of dying in store—2 to 1
6. In middle of crowd—chances of dying in store—10 to 1

Therapist: So. . .when you were in the crowd you thought you had a ten to one chance of dying.

Patient: It was crowded and stuffy and I couldn't catch my breath. I felt I was passing out. I really panicked and got out of there.

Therapist: What do you think—right now—were the actual probabilities that you would have died if you stayed in the store?

Patient: Probably one in a million.

The next time the patient went to the store her estimates of the probabilities of dying were much lower than during her previous trip. After further discussion, she was able to integrate the concept that a crowded store was not a threat to her life. As she entered the store, she reminded herself that she had already reached the conclusion—based on reason—that the store was a safe place. Subsequently, she experienced only trivial discomfort in stores and in other crowded places.

The pleasure-pain rules are similar to each other: One is often the converse of the other. Certain of these rules are so gross that they are completely at variance with reality or they have long-range results that interfere with some life objectives the patient values highly. An example of such an attitude: "It is wonderful to be famous." The converse, held by many people, is: "I can never be happy if I'm not famous." People who are dominated by these rules are constantly under the gun: driving themselves towards achieving prestige, popularity, or power; chalking up a point when they make a gain, subtracting points when they do not. The slavish following of these rules frequently interferes with other objectives such as living a reasonably healthy, tranquil life, having satisfying relationships with other people.

Even more crucial is the fact the certain people are likely to become depressed by overemphasizing these rules. The following sequence is seen among people as they go into a depression: Initially they judge that they are not making progress toward the evanescent goal—for example, fame. From this follows a series of deductions: "If I don't become famous, I have failed . . . I have lost the only thing that really matters . . . I am a failure . . . There's no point in going on . . . I might as well kill myself." When the patient examines the initial premise, he realizes that he has lost sight of gratifications other than being famous. He also realizes how he has boxed himself in by defining his own happiness in terms of fame. Similarly, people who define their happiness exclusively in terms of being loved by a particular person or persons set themselves up for fluctuations from happy to sad, depending on whether they regard themselves as loved or rejected. They, also, may be vulnerable to depression.

Some of the attitudes that predispose people to excessive sadness or depression are listed below:

1. In order to be happy, I have to be successful in whatever I undertake.
2. To be happy, I must be accepted (liked, admired) by all people at all times.
3. If I'm not on top, I'm a flop.
4. It's wonderful to be popular, famous, wealthy; it's terrible to be unpopular, mediocre.
5. If I make a mistake, it means that I'm inept.
6. My value as a person depends on what others think of me.
7. I can't live without love. If my spouse (sweetheart, parent, child) doesn't love me, I'm worthless.

8. If somebody disagrees with me, it means he doesn't like me.
9. If I don't take advantage of every opportunity to advance myself, I will regret it later.

Rules such as the above are likely to lead to misery. It is impossible for a person to be loved totally, at all times by all his friends. The degree of love and acceptance fluctuates considerably. The rules are framed in such a way, however, that any diminuation of love is likely to be regarded as a rejection.

Another problem posed by excessive reliance on acceptance, admiration, or love is that we do not possess a reliable gauge that another person is, indeed, rejecting, reproaching, or critical of us. As pointed out previously, we can verify objectively when somebody has attacked us physically by examining the site of the injury. But when somebody *seems* to be rejecting us, how do we know that we have not misinterpreted his behavior? Our subjective feelings of distress cannot be used to validate our interpretation because such feelings can occur whether the interpretation is right or wrong. This lack of validating information makes it immensely more difficult to deal with psychological trauma than physical injury.

A major technique of cognitive therapy consists of making the patient's attitudes explicit and helping him decide whether they are self-defeating. Moreover, it is essential that he learn from his own experience that because of certain attitudes he ends up with less happiness and more misery than if he were guided by more moderate or realistic rules. The therapist's role should be to suggest alternative rules for the patient's consideration—not to "brainwash" him.

Related to the pleasure-pain rules are the set of rules called the "tyranny of the shoulds" (Horney, 1950). If a person has the rule, "In order to be happy, I need to be loved by everybody," he is likely to implement this by another rule, "I should make everybody love me." The "shoulds" and "should nots" have a slave-driving quality and have much in common with Freud's conceptualization of the superego.

Some of the common "shoulds" are:

1. I should be the utmost of generosity, considerateness, dignity, courage, unselfishness.
2. I should be the perfect lover, friend, parent, teacher, student, spouse.
3. I should be able to endure any hardship with equanimity.
4. I should be able to find a quick solution to every problem.
5. I should never feel hurt; I should always be happy and serene.
6. I should know, understand, and foresee everything.
7. I should always be spontaneous; I should always control my feelings.
8. I should assert myself; I should never hurt anybody else.
9. I should never be tired or get sick.
10. I should always be at peak efficiency.

THE OVER-ALL STRATEGY

There are so many different therapeutic tactics available to the cognitive therapist that unless he develops an over-all strategy for a given case, the therapy may follow an erratic course based on trial and error. The principles that form the framework for cognitive therapy have been outlined previously in this chapter and also in the earlier chapters: clarifying the patient's distortions, self-injunctions, and self-reproaches that lead to his distress or disability, and helping him to revise the underlying rules that produce these faulty self-signals. Some of the methods used by the cognitive therapist are similar to those used previously by patients in their successful attempts at problem-solving. The therapist works with the patient in a more systematic way on psychological problems he has been unable to resolve independently. The specific mechanics consist of defining the problem areas precisely, filling in the informational gaps, establishing relations among the data, and forming generalizations. The therapist then helps the patient to use his own problem-solving apparatus in making the necessary adjustments in his ways of interpreting his experiences and regulating his behavior.

The *techniques* of psychotherapy overlap considerably with the *process* of psychotherapy, so that it is difficult to draw a line between what the therapist does and the patient's responses. Furthermore, the therapist may be employing several procedures simultaneously, and the patient may be reacting to these with a series of therapeutic responses. For instance, in training the patient to recognize his automatic thoughts, the therapist directly or indirectly questions their validity. In turn, the process of extending the patient's awareness of this form of ideation is accompanied by greater objectivity (distancing). As the patient recognizes that these self-signals are maladaptive or discordant with reality, he has a tendency to correct them automatically. Moreover, this kind of self-scrutiny leads directly to the recognition of the underlying premises and equations—the rules that are responsible for the faulty responses. The following case illustrates the interaction of the therapist's procedures and the patient's psychological processes.

An attractive young mother of three children was seen in a university psychiatric clinic because of episodes of anxiety lasting up to six or seven hours a day. These periods of anxiety had occurred practically daily for over four years. She had frequently consulted her family physician, who had prescribed a variety of sedatives and Thorazine, without any apparent improvement.

At the time of my first interview with her, the following facts were elicited. Her first anxiety episode occurred about two weeks after she had had a miscarriage. She was bending over to bathe her one-year-old son, when she suddenly began to feel faint. She then had her first anxiety attack, which lasted several hours. The patient could not find any explanation for her anxiety. When I asked whether she had had any thought at the time she felt dizzy, she recalled having had the idea, "Suppose I should pass out and injure the baby." It seemed plausible, as a working hypothesis, that her dizziness (which was probably the result of a postpartum anemia) led to the fear she might faint and drop the baby. This frightening notion produced anxiety, which she interpreted as a sign that she was "going to pieces."

Until the time of her miscarriage, the patient had been reasonably carefree and did not recall having experienced any episodes of anxiety. After her miscarriage, however, she periodically had the thought, "Bad things can happen to me." Subsequently, when she heard of someone becoming sick, she often would think, "This can happen to me," and she would begin to feel anxious.

The patient was instructed to try to pinpoint any thoughts that preceded further episodes of anxiety. At the next interview, she reported:

1. One evening, she heard that the husband of one of her friends had severe pneumonia. She immediately had an anxiety attack lasting several hours. In accordance with the instructions, she tried to recall the cognition preceding her anxiety. She remembered thinking, "Tom (her husband) could get sick like that and maybe die."

2. She had considerable anxiety just before leaving on a trip to her sister's house. She focused on her ideation and recognized that she had the repetitive thought, "I might get sick on the trip." She had had a serious episode of gastroenteritis during a previous trip to her sister's house and evidently believed that she was likely to get sick again.

3. On another occasion, she was feeling uncomfortable, and objects seemed somewhat unreal to her. She then had the thought, "I might be losing my mind," and immediately experienced an anxiety attack lasting almost an hour.

4. She learned that one of her friends had been committed to a state mental hospital. This bit of information led to the thought, "This could happen to me. I could lose my mind." When questioned about the specific details of losing her mind, she stated that she was afraid that if she went crazy, she would do something that would harm either her children or herself.

It was evident that the patient's major fears revolved around the anticipation of loss of control, whether by fainting or by becoming psychotic, and consequently doing something harmful. I explained to the patient that there was no evidence that she was becoming psychotic. She was also provided with an explanation for the arousal of her anxiety and of her secondary elaboration of the meaning of these attacks: Her underlying formula was that the symptoms of anxiety indicated she was on the verge of psychosis. During the next few weeks, her anxiety attacks became less frequent and less intense and, by the end of four weeks, they disappeared completely.

The major therapeutic thrust in this case was coaching the patient to recall the thoughts that preceded an anxiety attack and to assess their validity. The recognition that these attacks were initiated by a cognition rather than by some vague mysterious force convinced her that her notion that she was totally vulnerable was incorrect. She also realized that her belief that she was unable to control her reactions was erroneous. By learning to pinpoint the anxiety-producing thoughts, she was able to gain some detachment and to subject them to reality testing. Consequently, she was able to nullify the effects of those thoughts.

The formulation of the progress of this patient can now be fitted into the therapeutic model: (1) *self-observations* that led directly to the ideation preceding the anxiety; (2) establishing the relation between the thoughts and anxiety attack; (3) learning to regard thoughts as hypotheses rather than facts; (4) testing the hypotheses; (5) piecing together the assumptions that underlay and generated these hypotheses; (6) demonstrating that these rules composing her belief system were incorrect. Her belief system consisted of equations regarding probable mental and physical illness, loss of control, and involuntarily hurting somebody. Furthermore, she had developed the superstition that if something bad happened to someone else, it was likely to happen to her or a member of her family. Finally, she had developed the universal frightener, "Anything can happen to me." By demonstrating the fallacy of her equations and self-references, we were able to revise the faulty belief system.

CHAPTER 11

The Cognitive Therapy of Depression

> *If thou are pained by any external thing, it is not this thing that disturbs thee, but thine own judgment about it. And it is in thy power to wipe out this judgment now.*—Marcus Aurelius

RATIONALE OF THE COGNITIVE APPROACH

At various times, I have used most of the approaches to depression described in the contemporary literature. Particular methods seemed to help sometimes and to have an adverse effect at other times: expressing abundant warmth and sympathy, "getting out the anger," encouraging the patient to express sad or guilty feelings, interpreting his "need to suffer," urging him to be more self-accepting. However, talking about how miserable and hopeless they felt and trying to squeeze out anger often seemed to accentuate the patients' depression; their acceptance of their debased self-image and pessimism simply increased their sadness, passivity, and self-blame.

In the course of time, I found that tailoring a technique to selected characteristics of the depression syndrome as well as to the personality of the patient was far more effective than the previous approaches. Moreover, a highly structured, problem-oriented approach appeared to have more immediate results than the other methods. In addition, I found that specific cognitive and behavioral techniques were most effective in influencing mood and behavior.

In order to understand the cognitive approach to the treatment of depression, it is necessary to formulate the problems of the depressed patient in cognitive terms. The characteristics of depression can be viewed as expressions of an underlying shift in the depressed patient's cognitive organization. Because of the dominance of certain cognitive schemas, he tends to regard himself, his experiences, and his future in a negative way. These negative concepts are apparent in the way the patient systematically misconstrues his experiences and in the content of his ruminations. Specifically, he regards himself as a "loser." First, he believes that he has lost something of substantial value, such as a personal relationship, or that he has failed to achieve what he considers an important objective. Second, he expects the outcome of any activity he undertakes to be negative. Therefore, he is not motivated to set goals and, in fact, avoids engaging in "constructive" activities. Furthermore, he expects his entire future to be deficient in satisfactions, achievements. Third, he sees himself as a "loser" in the vernacular sense; he is inferior, inept, lacking in worth, awkward, and socially undesirable.

The patient's negative concepts contribute to the other symptoms of depression, such as sadness, passivity, self-blame, loss of pleasure response, and suicidal wishes. As a result of a vicious cycle, the negative thinking, unpleasant affects, and self-defeating motivations reinforce each other. The cognitive approach for counteracting depression consists of using techniques that enable the patient to see himself as a "winner" rather than a "loser," as masterful rather than helpless.

The cognitive approach involves, first of all, separating the syndrome of depression into its specific components. Conceivably, the therapist could start with any of the symptoms—emotional, motivational, cognitive, behavioral, or physiological—and concentrate his efforts on changing that symptom cluster. Each symptom cluster may be conceptualized as a problem and as a potential target for intervention. Since each of the components of depression contributes to other components, it might be anticipated that improvement in any one problem area would lead to improvement in others, and would finally spread to include the entire syndrome of depression.

The specific problems under consideration are complex and consist of more than the particular difficulty verbalized by the patient. A problem generally can be formulated in terms of three "levels": (a) The observable abnormal behavior or symptom, for example, easy fatigability, crying spells, suicidal threats; (b) the underlying motivational disturbances (if any), such as the wish to avoid activities or to escape from life; (c) underlying the motivation, a cluster of cognitions, such as the belief that striving toward a goal is futile, that there are no satisfactions ahead, and that he is defeated, deprived, and defective.

In each case, the selection of the specific problem and special techniques depends on a variety of factors. The therapist needs to sound out the patient and reach a consensus with the patient on which "target" problem to aim at and what methods to use. Generally, in the more severely depressed patient, a behavioral target, such as his inertia, is selected and special activity programs (for example, "Graded Task Assignment" or "Success Therapy") are set up. Of course, several targets and methods may be focused on concomitantly. A certain amount of trial-and-error and ingenuity is necessary. When the techniques have been selected, they must be adapted to the needs and personality of the patient.

The approach to a presenting symptom should encompass the less obvious components of the problem. For example, a project to mobilize the patient into activity not only involves increasing his motivation but also improving his self-esteem. The patient's own observation that he is successful in reaching a goal provides crucial information that affects his attitudes about himself.[1] As he thinks better of himself in terms of his ability to control his environment and to be effective in everyday situations, he begins to expect that the outcome of his efforts might be of some avail. Consequently, his optimism is increased. As has already been pointed out, an increase in positive expectancies improves motivation. The increased motivation leads to still better performance.

As the patient observes and correctly evaluates his improved performance, he is likely to experience an additional boost to his self-esteem. At the same time, he may begin to experience gratification from (a) the sense

[1]Bem (1967) and Wilkins (1971) have marshaled evidence that self-observations of behavior change lead to attitude change. A person drawing inferences from his overt behavior uses the same information that outside observers use in making judgments about his underlying attitudes.

of having accomplished something tangible and (b) the lifting of his self-esteem. One can see that a cycle has been completed through this particular maneuver: improved performance → elevation of self-esteem → increased motivation → improved performance. Any other element in the cycle, however, could potentially be used as a point of intervention.

The patient's perception of receiving a meaningful addition to his personal domain stimulates pleasant feelings. However, because of the depressive's tendency to downgrade or discredit positive happenings, he screens out many events that he would ordinarily construe as positive experiences. When the patient shows this tendency, his selective inattention should become the focus for discussion and then for application of a specialized technique.

In summary, then, the target approach consists of breaking up the problem of depression into component problems, selecting the specific multi-level problems to be attacked in a given case, and then determining what types of therapeutic intervention would be appropriate for the patient.

SYMPTOM, TECHNIQUE, AND MALADAPTIVE ATTITUDE

In formulating his approach to depression, it is important for the therapist to distinguish among symptom, technique, and underlying attitudes. For example, the symptom may be *affective,* such as crying spells, sadness, loss of gratification, loss of sense of humor, apathy. The therapeutic approach may be *behavioral,* for example, mobilizing the patient into more activity and positively reinforcing certain types of activity. The underlying attitude, however, is the component that needs to be changed ultimately if the totality of the depression is to be influenced. Thus, the goal is *cognitive modification.*

Engaging in activities leading to concrete successes (behavioral method) may help to counteract the attitude, "The future is hopeless because I cannot do anything constructive." Similarly, the negative cognitive set, "Everything is unpleasant," may be altered by visualizing pleasant scenes. Picturing pleasant scenes may also produce some gratification that can modify the individual's cognitive set to: "It is possible for me to experience some satisfactions rather than just continuous, unremitting pain" (Beck, 1967).

Merely focusing on the symptom (for example, sadness, wish to die, retarded behavior) without designing the program to include simultaneous attitude change may produce only temporary results. In fact, this "improvement" may be deceptive in that a single outward characteristic of depression is apparently changed, but the central core of the depression is not touched. A patient who is persuaded to engage in more activity may appear "better" but may then commit suicide. It is essential, therefore, that the therapist be alert to signs of fundamental attitude change as well as signs of symptomatic improvement.

Even though the mechanism of improvement is based on cognitive change, it is important to focus on a variety of targets, including those symptoms that are predominantly affective or motivational in nature. There are important reasons for using a multiple approach.

The direction of the downward spiral in depression can be reversed by modifying specific components of the chain reaction. For example, as a result of therapeutic instructions, a patient becomes more constructive. He observes his behavior and thinks, "I can do more things than I thought I could." This self-observation increases his motivation to expand his range of activities. As he reaches additional concrete goals, he experiences further improvement in his attitudes toward himself and toward the future. His improved self-image and increased optimism reduce his self-criticism and sadness, and he may, in fact, begin to experience some satisfactions. By designing his therapy in such a way as to affect several symptom groups simultaneously, the therapist can accelerate improvement.

It is crucial to recognize that simply inducing the patient to *act* less depressed does not mean that he *is* less depressed. A tubercular patient can be medicated to stop coughing and can be fattened with forced feeding so that he no longer looks emaciated. Yet cavities in his lungs remain just as large and caseous as ever. Similarly, a brain-damaged person may be trained to perform certain motor movements without their being any retrograde modification of his cerebral deficit. The proper assessment of improvement in depression requires an investigation of changes in affect, motivation, cognition, and physiological functions (sleep and appetite) as well as overt behavior.

THE MECHANICS OF COGNITIVE REORGANIZATION

Kelly's (1955) notion of the patient and the therapist as scientists who collaborate in investigating the patient's personal constructs is a useful analogy for understanding the technique of cognitive modification. The patient takes his assumptions or constructs so much for granted that he usually is unlikely to articulate them until he is pointedly questioned about them. The therapist helps the patient to make explicit the assumptions underlying his depression and then, working together, they scrutinize, probe, and test these assumptions.

Challenging the basic assumptions is important in treating patients, such as depressives, whose cognitive organization is essentially a "closed system." The system does not accommodate contradictory information. The postulates are accepted as facts. Improvement is related to opening the system to new information and different points of view. Moreover, the specific cognitive schemas become more elastic and permeable.

Through questioning, a particular assumption may be subjected to argument. The procedure consists of: (1) eliciting the patient's reasons for believing the depressogenic assumption, (2) marshaling, as in a debate, the evidence in favor of or contradictory to the assumption. The notion, as in the Socratic dialogues, is to find the "truth" through verbalizing the opposite position on a given issue.

Another important approach to testing the patient's beliefs is through empirical demonstration. It is possible for the two collaborators (therapist and patient) to set up an experimental situation in which the assumptions may be tested and an immediate answer can be obtained. We have carried out analog studies of this procedure with particular tasks and also have used a clinical derivation of these experimental paradigms in such clinical treatments as the Graded Task Assignment. *Success improved the performance of the depressed group,* whereas failure improved the performance of the nondepressed group (Loeb et al., 1971).

Our experimental finding that the depressed patient reacts positively to tangible evidence of successful or superior performance (Chapter 5), provides useful clues for cognitive restructuring. The meaning to the patient of immediate, concrete, positive information about his performance has a powerful effect on his self-concept and his expectancies. The tendency of the depressed patient to overgeneralize in a *positive* direction after "success" demonstrates that his negative cognitive set is malleable. The therapeutic application consists of devising techniques to pinpoint for the patient his specific cognitive distortions and to demonstrate their invalidity. By achieving such a cognitive reorganization through behavioral or interview techniques, the patient may experience rapid diminution in all the symptoms of his depression.

In the following sections, various approaches to the specific problem areas ("targets") will be described. A number of specialized techniques will be discussed. For purposes of clarity, a brief description of these techniques will be presented first.

Scheduling Activities with the Patient. Since the patient sees himself as ineffective, it is important for him to be active in order to observe himself as potentially more effective. An activity schedule, in itself, helps the patient to structure his day. Because depressed patients often resist attempts to get them to be "busy," it is essential to use a variety of incentives, such as the notion that being more active may relieve his unpleasant feelings to some degree.

Graded Task Assignment. The purpose of this method is to give the patient a series of successes and, therefore, is sometimes called "success therapy." The therapist starts with a simple assignment which he is able to determine is well within the patient's capability. Working together, therapist and patient design more activities along a complexity and duration gradient. For example, a depressed housewife initially might be encouraged simply to boil an egg. With each successive mastered experience, she can build up to preparing an entire meal.

Mastery and Pleasure Therapy [*M & P Therapy*]. The essence of this kind of therapy is to have the patient keep a running account of his activities and to mark down "M" for each mastery experience and "P" for each pleasure experience. The purpose of this procedure is to penetrate the "blindness" of depressed patients to situations in which they are successful and their readiness to forget situations that do bring them some satisfaction.

Cognitive Reappraisal. As noted previously, cognitive therapy utilizes a number of techniques whose major mode of action is the modification of faulty patterns of thinking. This technique consists essentially of identifying the typical maladaptive cognitions and attitudes. This ideation is then evaluated by patient and therapist to test its validity. There are at least seven steps: (1) identification of sequence between depressive cognitions and sadness; (2) identification of sequence between cognitions and motivations (avoidance wishes and suicidal impulses); (3) exploration of depressive cognitions; (4) examination, evaluation, and modification of these cognitions; (5) identification of overgeneralization, arbitrary inference, dichotomous thinking; (6) identification of underlying assumptions; (7) examination, evaluation and modification of basic premises and assumptions.

Alternative Therapy. This method consists of two different approaches: (1) Considering alternative explanations for experiences. The depressed patient shows a systematic negative bias in his interpretations. By thinking of other explanations, he is enabled to recognize his bias and to substitute more accurate interpretations. (2) Considering alternative ways of dealing with psychological and situational problems. By discussing different ways of dealing with his problems, the patient finds solutions to problems that he considered insoluble. He also realizes that options he has already discarded may be viable and can lead him out of his dilemma.

Cognitive Rehearsal. This technique is used to expose the problems that deter a patient from carrying out goal-directed activities. By imagining himself going through the steps involved in the specified activity, the patient is able to report the specific "obstacles" he anticipates and the conflicts that are aroused. These blocks to action can then be the focus of discussion.

Homework Assignments. It is apparent from the foregoing that the cognitive therapy of depression requires a substantial amount of work outside of the therapy hour. Homework assignments are made at each session. The patient is generally expected to carry out certain activities that will counteract his depressive symptoms. In addition, he usually keeps a log of automatic thoughts. The specific technique consists of writing down a negative cognition in one column and the rational response in another column. The specific problem areas and the recommended therapeutic techniques are delineated in Table 1.

TARGETS OF COGNITIVE MODIFICATION

TARGET: INERTIA, AVOIDANCE, FATIGABILITY

The typical passivity and apparent enervation in depression have been regarded historically as a form of neurophysiological inhibition: psychomotor retardation. However, numerous studies and clinical experience show that the patient becomes more active and performs effectively when his motivation is aroused by the experimenter or therapist (Loeb et al., 1971; Friedman, 1964). Hence, an activity schedule specifically devised for a given patient is warranted to counteract the apparent retardation.

There are many positive advantages from a rationally designed activity program. Some of these are: (a) The patient's self-concept is changed. He sees himself as more masterful and less inept. Concomitantly, with the improvement in his self-concept, he becomes more optimistic. (b) He is distracted from his painful, depressing thoughts and his painful affect by transferring his attention to the activity. (c) Other people's responses to the patient become more positive; "significant others" generally reinforce the patient's constructive activity in a beneficial way. (d) There may be a change in his affective response; he begins to enjoy the activities and thus feels better.

It is essential initially to create the motivation for the activity. Also the activity must have a rationale that is

TABLE 1
THE TARGET APPROACH TO DEPRESSION

Specific Problem Area (target)	Reasons Given by Patient	Therapeutic Approach
I. Behavioral Symptoms		
1. Inactivity	1. Too tired or weak	1. Probes
2. Withdrawal	2. Pointless to try	(a) What lost by trying?
3. Avoidance	3. Will feel worse if active	(b) Has passivity done any good?
	4. Will fail at anything I try	(c) Will feel worse if passive
		(d) How do you know?
		2. Activity schedule
		3. Graded task assignment
		4. Cognitive rehearsal

Table 1, continued

II. Suicidal Wishes		
	1. No point to living 2. Too miserable, need escape 3. Burden to others 4. Cannot cope with obligations/problems	1. Expose ambivalence (a) Question reasons for dying (b) List reasons for living 2. Alternative therapy (a) Alternative views of problems (b) Alternative actions 3. Reduce problem to manageable units
III. Hopelessness		
	1. Nothing will work out 2. Same as suicidal "reasons"	1. Empirical demonstration of fallacy of negative predictions 2. Question "reasons"

Table 1, continued

IV. Lack of Gratification	1. Cannot enjoy anything 2. No satisfactions 3. Activities do not mean anything	1. Remove "blinders" 2. M&P Therapy: *Look* for gratifications and label them 3. Explore meaning of goals 4. Counteract "killjoy thoughts"
V. Self-criticisms Self-hate	1. Am defective, weak, etc. 2. I *should* be more adequate 3. Am responsible for problems	1. Identify and reason with self-criticisms 2. Role-play: self-sympathy 3. Discuss: "tyranny of shoulds" 4. Triple column technique

Table 1, continued

VI. Painful Affect	1. I can't stand the pain 2. Nothing can make me feel better	1. Distraction 2. Raise threshold by ignoring affect 3. Counteract with humor, anger 4. Induced imagery 5. Triple column technique
VII. Exaggeration of External Demands, Problems, Pressures	1. I am overwhelmed 2. There is so much to do, I can never do it	1. Problem resolution (a) List things to do (b) Set priorities (c) Check off accomplished tasks (d) Concretize and split up external problems 2. Cognitive rehearsal

understandable—or can be made understandable—to the patient. Stimulating the motivation for activity requires a reasonable amount of understanding and skill on the part of the therapist. Anyone who has worked with depressed patients knows that they often make efforts to become more active. Moreover, their family and friends generally cajole, prod, or exhort them to be more active—without success. These efforts are generally abortive because the patient and those prodding him do not understand the psychology of depression.

In order to help mobilize a patient into activity, the therapist must first elicit the patient's reasons for his inactivity. In order to obtain this information, the therapist may recommend a particular activity or project that is obviously within the patient's capacity. When the patient expresses his reluctance or inability to accede to the suggestion, the therapist asks the patient to detail the reasons for his reluctance. These "reasons" are then treated as hypotheses to be tested by devising a specific project.

The usual reasons given by depressed patients for their passivity, inertia, and resistance to engaging in a project are: (a) "It is pointless to try." (b) "I cannot do it." (c) "If I try anything, it won't work out and I'll only feel worse." (d) "I am too tired to do anything." (e) "It is much easier to just sit still."

The patient generally accepts reasons for not being more active as valid, and it does not occur to him that they may be fallacious until after he has expressed them. Later, when the therapist designs an activity project with the patient, the validity of these "reasons" is tested. If the patient achieves the specified goal, the therapist should verify that the success experience contradicts the erroneous attitude (for example, that he is too weak to do anything).

Before the project is initiated, the meanings and connotations of the symptom should be explored and discussed. For instance, one of the connotations of being immobile is that the patient is "lazy." He tends to hold this point of view, as do the people around him. As a result, he criticizes himself—as do the significant others. By mobilizing the patient into activity, the therapist can help the patient to combat his pejorative self-evaluations.

The next stage in the cognitive-behavioral approach consists of engaging the patient's interest or curiosity so that he will at least cooperate to the extent of attempting a simple project. This can be accomplished through a novel presentation of a specific task, by explaining the rationale for the particular procedure, and by conveying to the patient the idea that there is a less painful alternative to feeling as bad as he does—namely, through collaborating with the therapist by involving himself in a specific activity. When the patient responds to the incentive to cooperate, then a variety of verbal cognitive or behavioral methods can be used.

Since the depressed patient's desire to escape from everyday activities is strong and his negative beliefs are entrenched, it is important for the therapist to state clearly to the patient how he is unwittingly defeating himself and making himself more miserable by blandly accepting his self-defeating attitudes and yielding to his regressive wishes. The therapist should indicate to the patient, directly or indirectly, that by questioning his ideas, he is likely to feel better.

It is crucial that the therapist pose his questions and assertions regarding the patient's self-defeating ideas and wishes in a nonjudgmental, reflective way. He should avoid the appearance of scolding the patient, and making him defensive. Because depressed patients generally respond to "criticism" with further self-criticisms and self-immobilization, the therapist should elicit the patient's reactions to his statements; he should determine whether the patient is using the therapist's comments "against himself."

The therapist, furthermore, should be vigilant lest his statements be construed simply as a summons to invoke "the power of positive thinking." He should indicate clearly that he and the patient are attempting to *pinpoint* a problem and provide a remedy for it. Global exhortations to "think positively" rarely help to correct unreasonable negative thinking and thus lead the patient to a further sense of failure.

After outlining his pragmatic approach, the therapist should encourage the patient to state his points of agreement and disagreement. This approach may seem fairly obvious and superficial, and one might reasonably wonder how it could be effective in counteracting the patient's powerful regressive wishes and negative ideas. In working with depressed patients, however, I have been impressed repeatedly by the degree to which they have accepted their avoidance wishes and nihilistic attitudes without examining them. By exposing these locked-in attitudes for examination and consideration, the therapist gives the patient an opportunity to modify them. An ultimate goal of this program is to train the patient to identify his negative thoughts without the immediate help of the therapist. As the patient recognizes how these automatic thoughts are defeating him, he may begin to challenge them spontaneously. At a later stage, he may correct them and substitute more rational responses (Chapter 10).

Some of the questions and statements I have found helpful in prompting a patient to examine—and then question—his beliefs are listed below. The therapist should not simply ask rhetorical questions but should give the patient time to respond to each question.

Patient: It is useless to try.

Therapist: You realize that you are not getting anywhere by being inactive. You have been doing this for a long time and you know that you are not feeling any better. What do you have to lose by experimenting with a different approach?

Patient: I will feel worse if I try to do something.

Therapist: (a) Do you feel that just lying around is going to make you feel any better? (b) Has your inactivity made you feel better up until now? (c) If being passive hasn't helped up until now, is there any reason why it should work now? (d) At least if you try some other pattern, you stand a chance of improvement. It is conceivable, of course, that you might feel worse, but one thing seems clear: If you lie around the way you have, there is little chance at all of your feeling better. (e) If you avoid activity you only criticize yourself and call yourself names such as lazy, inadequate, helpless. . . You have found that doing nothing keeps you preoccupied with your self-critical thinking. You lay yourself open to being victimized by these painful thoughts and feelings.

Patient: I can't do it.

Therapist: (a) How can you be so absolutely certain that you can't do this assignment unless you try?

(b) If you do a little bit at a time, you will be able to do it all.

Patient: I am too tired [or too sick] to try it.

Therapist: Once you get going, you may find that it is is easier to keep going than you realize. You will find you aren't too tired to keep at it. . . It takes tons of coal to get a train started, but very little to keep it going.

When the therapist is able to penetrate the patient's resistances and engage his interest, he then proceeds to the next stage in the therapeutic program. The therapist should not be content with simply producing cognitive dissonance, but must insure that whatever advantage is gained through discussion is followed immediately by action.

The therapeutic program may be formulated in terms of the following steps: (a) proposing a specific project to the patient; (b) eliciting his reasons for opposing the proposal; (c) asking the patient to weigh the validity of his "reasons" (or negative attitudes); (d) indicating to the patient why these reasons (or attitudes) are self-defeating and invalid; (e) stimulating the patient's interest in attempting to perform the proposed assignment; (f) setting up the project in such a way that the patient's performance will test the validity of his ideas. Thus, successful completion of the task will contradict the patient's hypothesis that he is incapable of doing it; (g) after the successful experience, indicating to the patient how the favorable outcome contradicts his self-defeating predictions; (h) reviewing with the patient the "constructive" attitudes proposed previously by the therapist. These formulations may be used later by the patient to combat his negative thoughts and attitudes; (i) training the patient in identifying negative thoughts, challenging them, and giving reasonable answers to them. This technique is implemented through homework assignments.

The patient uses three columns to write down (a) the situation that elicited unpleasant feeling, (b) the negative automatic thought, (c) the corrective response to the negative thought. How a patient's interest can be engaged by suggesting an activity that seems farfetched to him is illustrated in the following case excerpt:

The patient was a fifty-two-year-old man who had spent over a year in a hospital without moving away from his bed. He had had many trials of antidepressant medications without any improvement. I saw him for only one visit. At this time, the patient was sitting in a chair next to his bed. After preliminary introductions and general social interchanges, the interview proceeded thus:

> *Therapist:* I understand that you haven't moved away from your bedside for a long time. Why is that?
>
> *Patient:* I can't walk.
>
> *Therapist:* Why is that...Are your legs paralyzed?
>
> *Patient:* [irritated] Of course not! I just don't have the energy.
>
> *Therapist:* What would happen if you tried to walk?
>
> *Patient:* I'd fall on my face, I guess.
>
> *Therapist:* What would you say if I told you that you were capable of walking any place in the hospital?
>
> *Patient:* I'd say you were crazy.

Therapist: How about testing that out?

Patient: What's that?

Therapist: Whether I'm crazy.

Patient: Please don't bother me.

Therapist: You said you didn't think you could walk. Many depressed people believe that, but when they try it they find they do better than they expected.

Patient: I *know* I can't walk.

Therapist: Do you think you could walk a few steps?

Patient: No, my legs would cave in.

Therapist: I'll bet you can walk from here to the door [about 5 yards].

Patient: What happens if I can't do it?

Therapist: I'll catch you.

Patient: I'm really too weak to do it.

Therapist: Suppose I hold your arm. [The patient then took a few steps supported by the therapist. He continued to walk beyond the prescribed five yards—without further assistance. He then walked back to his chair, unassisted.]

Therapist: You did better than you expected.

Patient: I guess so.

Therapist: How about walking down to the end of the corridor [about 20 yards]?

Patient: I know I don't have the strength to walk that far.

Therapist: How far do you think you can walk?

Patient: Maybe, to the next room [about 10 yards].

The patient easily walked to the next room and then continued to the end of the corridor. The therapist continued to propose specific goals and to elicit the patient's responses to the goals. After successful completion of each task, a greater distance was proposed.

Within 45 minutes, the patient was able to walk freely around the ward. He was thereby able to "reward" himself for his increased activity by being able to obtain a soda from the vending machine. Later, when he extended the range of his activities, he was able to walk to different points in the hospital and gain satisfaction from various recreational activities. Within a few days, he was playing ping-pong and going to the hospital snack bar and, in less than a week, he was able to walk around the hospital grounds and enjoy seeing the flowers, shrubs, and trees. Another automatic reward was the favorable response he received from members of the hospital staff and from the other patients. The patient began to speak about himself in positive terms and to make concrete plans for leaving the hospital permanently—a goal he reached in a month.

This case illustrates how it is possible to break through a patient's negative beliefs. After a successful experience, his view of himself changes—from being sick, weak, subhuman—to being a functioning human being, able to move himself to sources of satisfaction. If the patient had not shown a shift in his self-regard and expectancies, it would have been crucial to point out to him how his actual performance contradicted his negative views and, therefore, warranted a more positive concept.

In more complex assignments, the therapist must realize that the patient will have negative thoughts in reference to each step of the task. The patient must be properly prepared to cope with these negative thoughts and to counteract them. For example, a patient was given the assignment to fix his phonograph. In planning the specific steps in this project, he had negative thoughts that discouraged him (for example, "I won't be able to find the screwdriver"). These thoughts were expressed by the patient and discussed ("Where do you generally keep the screwdriver?"). After the discussion succeeded in cutting through the self-defeating thoughts, the next step in the project and the accompanying negative thoughts were discussed. As a result of this cognitive rehearsal, the patient was able to implement the plan and thus not only gain the satisfaction of having accomplished a task he considered impossible, but also the pleasure of being able to listen to his records.

TARGET: HOPELESSNESS AND SUICIDAL WISHES

When asked why he wants to commit suicide, the patient usually responds: (a) "There is no point to living. I have nothing to look forward to." (b) "I am feeling so miserable and this is the only way I can escape." (c) "I am a burden to my family and I can help them by removing myself." (d) "The future is black." (e) "I can't get what I want anyhow so what's the use of trying."

Note that all of these attitudes obviously are related to hopelessness. The patient typically regards himself as locked into an insoluble life situation from which there is no escape (except by suicide). If hopelessness is at the core of the suicidal wishes, a variety of methods can be used to convey to the patient that there are (a) alternative interpretations of his life situation and different interpretations of his future, and (b) that he has other choices than his current behavior, which is leading to a blind alley. We have dubbed this approach "alternative therapy."

The therapist should not evade probing for the reasons the patient regards suicide as the only escape from his misery or intolerable life situation. The patient generally has considered alternative solutions but has discarded them as useless. The therapist should re-examine these alternatives with the patient. Often, the patient has decided on suicide because he has concluded that he cannot be helped or that his life situation cannot be changed. By examining his basic assumptions, the patient may be guided to shift the balance between life-preservative wishes and self-destructive wishes.

A teen-age girl reported that her future looked pretty grim and she was seriously considering suicide. She stated as her reason for suicide that she had felt unhappy during most of her childhood and that, "Childhood is supposed to be the happiest period of your life." Thus, she could only look ahead to increased unhappiness as she grew older. I was able to discuss with her that most people I knew claimed that they were happier in their adulthood than in their childhood. The patient was surprised to hear this.

She also asserted that her future was bleak for her because she was not attaining the high standards that she had set for herself in her art work. She was amused when I pointed out to her that many people, including me, could not even draw a straight line and yet were happy. She was willing to consider setting more flexible standards for herself. Moreover, she was able to see that it was unwise to apply her subjective judgment of her performance to the over-all judgment of the value of life. More to the point, I indicated how she had identified herself with her work. Thus, if her work was a failure, *she* was a failure.

After this single discussion, she revamped her thinking. Several years later she told me that she had not had any recurrence of her hopelessness or suicidal wishes.

The assumptions underlying hopelessness and suicidal tendencies can be subtly undermined by skillful questions. By pointed, but friendly, questioning, the therapist can make the patient aware of the incongruity of some of his assumptions. Recognition of the incongruity helps to shake his faulty belief system. As a minimal goal, the questioning should be directed to encourage the patient to see that his assumptions are *ideas* that can be examined rather than indisputable reality or unshakeable *facts*.

An example of how a patient may become aware of the logical inconsistencies in his belief system is presented in the following interchange with a woman who had made a recent suicide attempt and still wanted to commit suicide. She had nothing to look forward to since her husband was unfaithful. The therapeutic technique is illustrated below.

Therapist: Why do you want to end your life?

Patient: Without Raymond, I am nothing. . . I can't be happy without Raymond. . . But I can't save our marriage.

Therapist: What has your marriage been like?

Patient: It has been miserable from the very beginning. . . Raymond has always been unfaithful. . . I have hardly seen him in the past five years.

Therapist: You say that you can't be happy without Raymond. . . Have you found yourself happy when you are with Raymond?

Patient: No, we fight all the time and I feel worse.

Therapist: You say you are nothing without Raymond. Before you met Raymond, did you feel you were nothing?

Patient: No, I felt I was somebody.

Therapist: If you were somebody before you knew Raymond, why do you need him to be somebody now?

Patient: [Puzzled] Hmmm...

Therapist: Did you have male friends before you knew Raymond?

Patient: I was pretty popular then.

Therapist: Why do you think you will be unpopular without Raymond now?

Patient: Because I will not be able to attract any other man.

Therapist: Have any men shown an interest in you since you have been married?

Patient: A lot of men have made passes at me, but I ignore them.

Therapist: If you were free of the marriage, do you think that men might be interested in you—knowing that you were available?

Patient: I guess that maybe they would be.

Therapist: Is it possible that you might find a man who would be more constant than Raymond?

Patient: I don't know...I guess it's possible.

Therapist: You say that you can't stand the idea of losing the marriage. Is it correct that you have hardly seen your husband in the past five years?

Patient: That's right, I only see him a couple of times a year.

Therapist: Is there any chance of your getting back together with him?

Patient: No...He has another woman. He doesn't want me.

Therapist: Then what have you actually lost if you break up the marriage?

Patient: I don't know.

Therapist: Is it possible that you'll get along better if you end the marriage?

Patient: There is no guarantee of that.

Therapist: Do you have a *real marriage?*

Patient: I guess not.

Therapist: If you don't have a real marriage, what do you actually lose if you decide to end the marriage?

Patient: [Long pause] Nothing, I guess.

Following this interview, the patient was more cheerful and it appeared that she was over the suicide crisis. In a subsequent interview, she stated that the point that really struck home was: How could she be "nothing" without Raymond—when she had lived happily and was an adequate person before she ever knew him? She eventually was divorced and settled down to a more stable life.

In this case, the "alternative therapy" was based on questioning the patient's faulty beliefs that (a) she needed her husband in order to be happy, function, or to have an identity; (b) that, somehow, the end of the marriage would be the end of the road for her, that it would be a devastating loss; and (c) she could have no future life without her husband. The patient was able to see the fallacy of her beliefs and consequently realized she had options besides either trying to preserve a dead marriage or committing suicide. In other cases, the realistic alternatives to self-destructive courses of action need to be specified by the therapist.

The role of hopelessness as a key factor in serious suicide attempts and suicidal ideation has been substantiated in a number of systematic studies (Minkoff, Bergman, Beck, and Beck, 1973; Lester and Beck, 1975; Beck, Kovacs, and Weissman, 1975; Wetzel, 1976). The psychotherapeutic value of focusing directly on the patient's *reasons* for wanting to commit suicide has also been indicated in a systematic study (Kovacs, Beck, and Weissman, 1975).

In using "alternative therapy," the therapist must bear in mind that the patient has a thick layer of pessimism enveloping any constructive alternatives that may be suggested. Since the patient regards his options in a negatively distorted way, the therapist must be wary not to accept the patient's blanket rejection of a plan at face value. The choice of suicide as a means of escape is often based on an unrealistically negative appraisal of the prognosis for other forms of escape (for example, medication, hospitalization, vacation, temporary leave of absence).

TARGET: SELF-CRITICISMS AND SELF-BLAME

The depressed patient, in common with other people, attempts to determine the cause of his problems. In his notion of causality, the depressed patient is prone to regard himself as the cause of his difficulties. He may carry this notion of self-causality to seemingly absurd extremes: When it is pointed out that self-blame is maladaptive, he then blames himself for blaming himself. The self-criticisms take the form of statements such as, "I am no good; I am a failure; it's my own fault." Of course, these ideas only make the patient feel worse.

The cognitive approach to self-criticisms consists, first, of making the patient aware of the steady stream of self-criticisms. This is generally not difficult because the patient usually feels worse after a self-criticism; thus, when he experiences a spurt of dysphoria, he need only "play back" his preceding thoughts to identify the self-criticism.

The next step is to increase the patient's objectivity toward his self-hate. This step is crucial since the patient commonly believes his self-criticism is justified. One method is to ask the patient a question such as, "Suppose I made mistakes the way you do? Would you despise me for it?" Inasmuch as the patient recognizes that he would not be so critical of another person, he may realize the exaggerated nature of his self-criticisms. Mildly to moderately depressed patients may recognize the self-defeating nature of their self-criticisms if the therapist says, for example, "How do you think I would perform if somebody were standing over my shoulder evaluating or criticizing everything I did?...In a sense, this is what you are doing without deliberately wanting to ...The net effect, however, is that you not only feel bad, but you can't perform adequately. You will find that you can be free with yourself and more successful if you try to ignore the self-evaluations."

The process of gaining objectivity towards the irrationality and self-destructiveness of the self-criticisms may sometimes be accelerated through role playing. The therapist, for example, plays the role of the patient as he sees himself: inadequate, inept, weak. The patient is coached to assume the role of a harsh critic who will verbally attack the "patient" for any demonstration or acknowledgement of a fault. A skillful therapist may play the role in such a way as to demonstrate the patient's distortions and arbitrary inferences. If the patient is properly "warmed up" to the critic role, he can simultaneously act out the denunciations and observe the extravagance of the negative judgments.

The self-criticisms can be attacked directly by training the patient to recognize the automatic thoughts edged with self-depreciation. The patient learns to challenge the validity of these negative thoughts and to substitute a more reasonable appraisal of himself. The "triple column" technique, referred to previously, enables the patient to pinpoint his negative thought and to specify why it is erroneous or maladaptive. Such homework assignments are crucial to implementing the strategies formulated during the therapeutic interview.

—

TARGET: PAINFUL AFFECT

Because of the intensity of the psychic pain in depression, it is important to alleviate the patient's sadness and other affective disturbances as soon as possible. Depressed patients frequently report that none of their usual sources of gratification brings them pleasure any more. In Costello's terms (1972), the patient has experienced "loss of reinforcer effectiveness."

Through a variety of techniques, it is possible to induce the patient to feel sorry for himself, cry, or be genuinely amused. Such experiences may help to thaw out his frozen affect. "De-icing" the frozen affect is a crucial technique in the treatment of severe depression. Encouraging a patient to express his unpleasant emotions through verbalizing them or crying sometimes reduces their intensity and makes the patient feel more alive, more like "a whole person." (Of course, some patients feel worse after emotional release; hence, such methods should be used with caution.)

When a patient cries, he may feel sympathy for himself. Thus, his cognitive set toward himself changes from rejecting or derogatory to sympathetic. Sympathy with oneself is inconsistent with the cognitive set of self-blame.

Feeling sorry for oneself can be analogized to the kind of empathy one experiences with characters who are portrayed as wronged or unfortunate in a movie. The people in the audience become dewy-eyed or sob because they *care* about the unfortunate character. Similarly, by feeling genuine pity for themselves, depressed patients are likely to be less self-critical (Efran, 1973). The process can be accelerated by a number of techniques. Telling the patient a story of another unfortunate person with a similar problem and with whom the patient can identify frequently evokes sympathy in the patient. Feeling sympathy for another person in the same situation helps the patient to regard himself sympathetically. Dramatic techniques such as role-playing, in which the therapist assumes the role of his depressed patient, may also help the patient to change his cognitive set from critical to sympathetic.

Some therapists are particularly skillful in eliciting amusement. Such a response may be evoked by the therapist's demonstrating the ironical aspects of a situation. Depressed patients who do not respond to usual kinds of humor may nonetheless retain their sensitivity to irony. The experience of amusement may be a temporary antidote to sadness because it involves a shift to a cognitive set that is not compatible with self-blame and deadly serious pessimism.

In mild or moderate depressions, the expression of anger by the patient may serve to shake loose positive affect—probably because it helps to change his cognitive set from self-blaming to other-blaming. It is likely that the patient begins to regard himself as a more effective person when he expresses anger. Being angry is not only more pleasant than being sad, but has connotations of power, superiority, and mastery. Modulated expression of anger often is a potent way of controlling or changing the behavior of other people. Thus, the expression of anger has cognitive consequences: The patient perceives himself in a more favorable way. Nonetheless, the expression of anger is often regarded negatively by the patient and may provoke other people; thus, it is not a reliable vehicle for improvement.

Finally, techniques may be used to raise the patient's threshold for his dysphoria. For example, the therapist and significant others may distract the patient from examining and monitoring his sad feelings by engaging him in some potentially interesting activity. The selection of an activity cannot be arbitrary, but requires collaborative planning and, often, considerable ingenuity.

The therapist may emphasize to the patient that it is possible to raise his threshold for psychic pain by ignoring the unpleasant feelings. The therapist may also point out that the unpleasant feeling tends to build up to a peak and then diminish. When the unpleasant feeling is peaking, the patient can predict that it will probably diminish before long. The ability to predict even temporary relief from dysphoria reduces the sense of helplessness and vulnerability. The expectation of even temporary respite makes the pain more bearable.

Mastery and Pleasure Therapy. Another important target is lack of gratification. The loss of "reinforcer effectiveness" may be explained in theoretical terms: Because of the patient's negative cognitive set, it is difficult for him to attach a positive meaning to his experiences. Nonetheless, there is clinical evidence that the depressed patient actually has more pleasurable experiences than he is able to recall or report when questioned (Rush, Khatami, and Beck, 1975). The selectivity of his recall is produced by an attitude such as, "I never enjoy anything anymore." This attitude is fortified by his failure to integrate his enjoyable experiences. Thus, his enjoyments are momentary, and the controlling memories consist of unpleasant experiences. When the patient is willing to record systematically the events of the day and to rate them according to the degree of satisfaction experienced, it is generally found that he has many more pleasant experiences than he had expected.

A number of techniques are available to sensitize a patient to positive experiences. The therapist can use the help of a significant other to recall pleasant events. We have found, for example, that a spouse is able to report recent pleasant events that the patient acknowledged as being pleasurable at the time, but was unable to recall later without help. The recollection during the interview session substantially improves the patient's mood (Rush, Khatami, and Beck, 1975).

Another technique consists of having the patient keep an hourly record of his waking activities. We have asked the patients to rate these activities according to the degree of pleasure evoked and, also, according to the degree of mastery involved. We have found that, as the patients realize the number of actual experiences of mastery or pleasure, they begin to feel a more enduring sense of satisfaction. Recognizing, labeling, and recalling mastery experiences are especially important in improving the patient's sense of competence and ability to cope. By attempting to deal with troublesome problems, the patient mobilizes his coping powers. If he can then integrate the successful experiences through the systematic coding techniques, he can consolidate a more positive self-image. Mastery experiences can be formulated within a program of graded task assignments.

A withdrawn, depressed student, in collaboration with the therapist, compiled a list of projects graded according to the amount of difficulty or stress they imposed. For example, during the first week he was "assigned" projects in an ascending order of difficulty: (a) buy books for his courses at the bookstore; (b) study in library for one hour a day; (c) telephone several old friends for a chat; (d) outline an overdue paper; (e) do the necessary library research for the paper; (f) write first draft of paper.

Although these projects might seem commonplace, completing them successfully represented a series of triumphs for the patient who experienced the first gratifications he had had in a long time.

The therapist may attempt to bring more gratification into a patient's life by listing activities that had been gratifying prior to the depression but which the patient had abandoned. Lewinsohn (1974b) used a computer to select ten activities that correlated most highly with the patient's good moods and then granted the patient increased therapy time in proportion to the time spent in these pleasant activities. He thus used therapy time as a reward for increasing activity levels.

The "rewards" for engaging in graded tasks can be administered by a friend or relative, who gives the patient praise and approval for successful completion of assignments (Gathercole, 1972). Explicit self-reinforcement may also enhance the value of graded task assignments. The patient may reinforce himself by scoring goal attainments with "A" on his daily log of activities (Rush, Khatami, and Beck, 1975) or by praising himself, doing something he likes, or giving himself a symbolic reward such as dispensing a designated number of poker chips (Jackson, 1972).

Leading the patient to review his life history with specific attention to successful and pleasurable experiences is often helpful. The patient—and therapist—are sometimes startled to find that the patient had a relatively successful and pleasant life prior to his depression. However, because of his negative cognitive set, he may have excluded the positive experiences in his global reconstructions of the past.

Past episodes representing mastery or pleasure may be revivified through the use of imagery techniques. The patient is instructed to imagine specific positive episodes as though they were occurring in the present, so that he may recapture the pleasant affect involved in the actual episode. Other imagery techniques also have been used to counteract the patient's tendency to construe events in an unpleasant way. The technique of "time projection" (Lazarus, 1968; Beck, 1970c) has been used to provide greater perspective on a current "traumatic" situation.

When he is upset about a current situation, the patient is instructed to visualize the situation at intervals in the future. When the problem is visualized from the perspective of the future, it often shrinks to appropriate proportions.

Although induced fantasy techniques are not applicable to every case of depression, they are often helpful. In some cases, the repeated imaging of a traumatic event may alleviate the associated distress. In other cases, expectations of future disaster may be reduced to realistic proportions by repeated visualization of the anticipated event (Beck, 1967).

EXAGGERATION OF EXTERNAL DEMANDS

Many depressed patients have a sense of being overwhelmed by the everyday problems of living. Certain responsibilities that were regarded as interesting challenges during the nondepressed period now seem to be impossible burdens. Some patients may feel so crushed by these "overwhelming burdens" that they think of suicide as the only way to escape. When the problems are discussed, however, it becomes apparent that the patient has greatly exaggerated their magnitude and importance. Through rational exploration, the patient may regain his perspective and then set about defining what has to be done and how to go about doing it. The therapist generally has to take the lead in helping the patient to list his responsibilities, set priorities, and formulate the appropriate course of action.

Since the implementation of the plan may be blocked by self-defeating thoughts, the therapist should use the kind of cognitive rehearsal described previously in order to elicit these negative thoughts. For instance, a depressed housewife felt paralyzed at the thought of marketing. After compiling a shopping list with the patient, the therapist suggested that she fantasize going to the supermarket. In her fantasy, she was stymied by indecision each time she attempted to select an item. It was discovered that the indecisiveness resulted from a stream of thoughts that she would make the wrong decision. When these self-doubts were dealt with in the therapy hour, she was able to have a fantasy of successfully making each purchase on her shopping list. She felt much more optimistic and, indeed, succeeded in doing her marketing in reality.[2]

OUTCOME STUDIES OF COGNITIVE AND BEHAVIORAL THERAPY

Three patients with chronic and relapsing depression were treated with a combination of cognitive and behavioral techniques. The main behavioral modality consisted of the use of activity schedules. The cognitive approach was directed at exposing and correcting the patients' negative distortions of the activities undertaken. These patients, although not substantially helped by drug therapy, showed prompt and sustained improvement with cognitive-behavioral therapy as reflected by their scores on the Hamilton and Beck depression measures (Rush, Khatami, and Beck, 1975).

Recent innovations in the behavior therapy of depression also consist primarily of highly structured and directive techniques (see Beck and Greenberg, 1974, for a

[2]This case and the induced fantasy technique are discussed in greater detail in Beck (1967), pp. 329-330.

review of the literature on cognitive and behavioral techniques). A number of case reports, analog and theoretical studies have supported the use of cognitive or behavioral techniques (Beck, 1974; Lewinsohn, 1974b; Lewinsohn and Atwood, 1969; Lewinsohn, Shaffer and Libet, 1969; Lewinsohn and Shaw, 1969; Lewinsohn, Weinstein, and Alper, 1970; Seitz, 1971; Wahler and Pollio, 1968). Quantitative outcome studies with follow-ups, however, have rarely been reported (Rardin and Wetter, 1972). The need for further refinement of therapeutic techniques has been underscored by recent reports indicating that supportive psychotherapy is relatively ineffective compared to antidepressant drugs in relieving the symptoms of depression (Klerman and Weissman, 1974).

A controlled study by Taylor (1974) offers substantial encouragement for the further development of cognitive and behavioral techniques. He provided several therapeutic approaches to college-student volunteers who had high scores on depression scales. Seven subjects were in each group. Each student received two treatments a week over a period of three weeks. Mildly to moderately depressed patients receiving *either* cognitive therapy or behavior therapy improved significantly more than did a waiting-list control group. Furthermore, the *combination* of cognitive and behavioral therapy was significantly more effective than either treatment alone.

A quantitative study by Shaw (1974) indicates the efficacy of cognitive therapy in a clinic population. He applied cognitive techniques to depressed patients who had been referred to a psychiatric outpatient clinic by family physicians after conventional therapy had failed. He treated the patients in individual psychotherapy twice a week for a total of 10 sessions. By the end of the fifth week, there was a significant improvement in six out of seven patients and follow-up at 10 weeks indicated that the mean depression scores were within the minimal depressed range.

Shaw (1975) obtained similar results in a controlled study using three types of group therapy with a population of college students who had sought help for depression at the student health clinic. He randomly assigned eight patients each to a cognitive therapy group, a behavior therapy group, a nondirective therapy group, and a waiting-list control group. The therapy groups met for two-hour sessions twice a week for four weeks (total, eight sessions). On post-test measures, the patients in the therapy groups were found to have improved significantly more than those on the waiting list. The cognitive therapy group showed almost twice as much improvement on the Depression Inventory (from 29.0 to 12.2) as the behavior therapy group (from 26 to 17), a difference that was statistically significant.

Our research group at the University of Pennsylvania has conducted a series of studies testing the efficacy of cognitive psychotherapy for chronically or intermittently depressed suicidal outpatients. Two systematic studies used psychiatric residents as therapists. The patients had intractable unipolar depressions. The average time since their first depression was eight years, and the median duration of the current episode was six months. All the patients had unsatisfactory response to treatment prior to referral to our clinic. In our first study of 23 patients treated by six psychiatric residents for a maximum 20 visits for a maximum of 20 weeks, we found that the improvement rate for those who remained in treatment was 70 per cent. On the basis of our experience, we determined that more frequent visits over a shorter period of time might produce better results.

The next study, which involved 31 outpatients, was designed as a controlled comparison of our psychotherapy with an antidepressant drug of proven efficacy (imipramine). In contrast to the first study, the patients in this study were seen twice a week for a maximum of 12 weeks. The frequency of visits tapered off toward the end of treatment. There were several interesting findings:

1. The psychotherapy and chemotherapy groups showed similar and prompt response to treatment. At the end of 12 weeks, 10 out of 12 psychotherapy cases had recovered; one was markedly improved, and one was moderately improved. The psychotherapy group did not show any dropouts from treatment, whereas five out of 18 chemotherapy patients discontinued treatment because of side effects or for other reasons.

2. Patients in the psychotherapy group showed more rapid improvement in the degree of hopelessness than did the drug-treated patients. Because hopelessness is an index of suicide risk, it is possible that this psychotherapy was more effective than chemotherapy in shortening the period of suicide risk.

3. During the first six weeks of treatment, patients in twice-a-week therapy improved twice as rapidly as the once-a-week patients in our first study.

4. At six months' follow-up, the psychotherapy patients maintained their improvement and their clinical progress was better than that of the drug-treated patients. (Rush, Beck, et al., 1975).

In summary, a wide variety of techniques are available for the modification of cognitive distortions and underlying maladaptive attitudes. Recent controlled outcome studies demonstrate the efficacy of these techniques and provide promise for the development and general acceptance of an empirically based psychotherapy for depressed patients.

CHAPTER 12

The Status of Cognitive Therapy

All crises begin with the blurring of a paradigm and the consequent loosening of the rules for normal research. . . A crisis may end with the emergence of a new candidate for paradigm and with the ensuing battle over its acceptance.—Thomas S. Kuhn

EVALUATING PSYCHOTHERAPIES: SOME CRITERIA

In view of the plethora of psychotherapies, is there room for cognitive therapy? How well do currently popular systems of psychotherapy meet existing standards? Does cognitive therapy represent an advance in the evolution of the psychotherapies, or is it simply another mutation destined for early extinction?

Before starting to evaluate the psychotherapies, we should distinguish between a system of psychotherapy and a simple cluster of techniques. A system of psychotherapy provides both a format for understanding the psychological disorders it purports to treat and a clear blueprint of the general principles and specific procedures of treatment. A well developed system provides (a) a comprehensive theory or model[1] of psychopathology and (b) a detailed description of and guide to therapeutic techniques related to this model.

STANDARDS FOR EVALUATING THEORIES OF PSYCHOPATHOLOGY

1. The theory should satisfy the requirements of any good scientific theory, namely, that it explain the phenomena within its domain with minimal complexity. According to the law of parsimony, the best theory accounts for the most data—and uses the simplest concepts. Moreover, the theory should be relatively free of internal contradictions, and its basic assumptions and hypotheses should be logically consistent with each other.

2. The theory of psychopathology should be closely related to its allied psychotherapy so that it is obvious how the psychotherapeutic principles are logically derived from the theory.

3. The theory should provide the basis for understanding why its derived psychotherapeutic techniques are effective. The rationale and mode of operation of the therapy should be implicit in the theory. In other words, the theory should provide more satisfactory explanations for the therapeutic effect than alternative theories. The history of medicine is replete with examples of effective therapies based on incorrect theories or superstitions.

4. The theory should be elastic enough to allow for development of new techniques without being so loose or

[1]For the purposes of this discussion, no clear distinction is made between "theory" and "model." A comprehensive description of the attributes of a good theory is presented by Epstein (1973).

complex that it obligingly dispenses a justification for any procedure a therapist might feel inspired to improvise.

5. An important challenge to a scientific model is the degree to which it is based on verified evidence. A related attribute is the degree to which its assumptions, axioms, and hypotheses can be tested through systematic investigations and experiments.

STANDARDS FOR EVALUATING SYSTEMS OF PSYCHOTHERAPY

1. The system of psychotherapeutic procedures should be well defined and clearly and explicitly described.

2. The general principles of treatment should be sufficiently well articulated so that different therapists dealing with the same problem among similar patients can be expected to use similar techniques. Furthermore, the blueprint of therapy should be sufficiently clear and comprehensive so that the neophyte therapist is not forced to proceed like an automaton following the same pat formula for each patient.

3. There should be empirical evidence to support the validity of the principles underlying the therapy. If, for example, a therapy is based on the technique of "reliving" an alleged traumatic episode in childhood or infancy, there should be evidence that (a) such an episode actually occurred; (b) it was traumatic; (c) it is currently contributing to the patient's problem; and (d) re-experiencing the episode enables the patient to solve his current problem.

4. The efficacy of the treatment should have empirical support, such as: (a) analog studies in which certain procedures identical to or analogous to those used

in therapy are applied to experimental subjects under highly controlled conditions; (b) carefully investigated single cases in which quantitative measures are used to demonstrate improvement at various stages of the treatment and at follow-up; (c) well-designed therapeutic trials, including quantitative measures, control groups, ratings by independent judges, and long-term follow-ups. In view of the well-known phenomena of spontaneous remission and "cures" based on suggestion, we need more than the claims of the therapist or testimonials from his patients in order to judge the value of a therapy.

Only a few of the popular therapies on the current scene meet the minimal requirements for a system of psychotherapy. Rogerian, or client-centered, therapy is reasonably specific in its prescribed procedures but explicitly avoids a comprehensive model of psychopathology (Rogers, 1951). The therapeutic techniques are intimately related to its few theoretical postulates; the principles of the therapy and of the model are readily testable. A number of outcome studies suggest that, for certain disorders at least, this form of therapy has beneficial effect.

Other therapies that have attracted considerable public attention have a weak empirical and theoretical basis. Transactional analysis (Berne, 1961), Gestalt therapy (Perls et al., 1951), primal therapy (Janov, 1970), and reality therapy (Glasser, 1965), show the same limitations: A theory of psychopathology is either skimpy or totally lacking; experimental evidence to support the principles of theory or therapy is not provided; and there have been no well-designed studies to demonstrate the efficacy of the particular methods used. Consequently, these therapeutic approaches are not sufficiently developed to fulfill the requirements of a system of psychotherapy.

In contrast, cognitive therapy, psychoanalysis, and behavior therapy (to a lesser extent, client-centered psychotherapy as well) do meet the criteria for a system of psychotherapy. While the theory and techniques of cognitive therapy have been presented previously in this volume, this chapter will examine the empirical basis for the cognitive approach. Cognitive therapy will be compared with psychoanalysis and behavior therapy. Finally, the current status of cognitive therapy as a system of psychotherapy will be evaluated.

THE COGNITIVE SYSTEM OF THERAPY

The cognitive model of psychopathology and the principles of cognitive therapy related to this model have been subjected to a number of empirical studies. Although considerable further research will be required to validate all aspects of the theory and of the therapy, the work to date supports many aspects of the theory.[2]

A central feature of the theory is that the content of a person's thinking affects his mood. A number of studies show that inducing a subject to focus on ideas of a self-enhancing or self-deflating content (for example, Velten, 1967; Coleman, 1970) produces feelings of elation or sadness respectively.

The concept that meaning determines the emotional response to a situation is supported by Pastore (1950,

[2]Mahoney (1974) has reviewed over 400 studies that directly or indirectly support the theoretical underpinnings of cognitive therapy. An even more extensive bibliography has been compiled by Ellis and Murphy (1975).

1952). He shows that the meaning attributed to a frustrating agent, rather than the frustration *per se,* is responsible for the arousal of anger. Similarly, Lazarus and his co-workers (1966) demonstrate that the conceptualization of the same situation as either threatening or innocuous leads respectively to anxiety or to a neutral response.

Studies of persons with anxiety in particular situations demonstrate how the self-signals or automatic thoughts contribute to the arousal of anxiety. For example, Meichenbaum, Gilmore, and Fedoravicius (1971) not only demonstrate the role of automatic thoughts in producing speech anxiety, but show that speech anxiety is reduced by cognitive therapy. Meichenbaum extends his findings to other problems, including text anxiety and phobias. Other investigators have established the role of negative thinking in producing anxiety in students apprehensive of tests (Liebert and Morris, 1967; Marlett and Watson, 1968). Similarly, Horowitz and his coworkers (1971) demonstrate the compulsive intrusion of automatic thoughts following stress.

Our own research studies have shown the influence of cognitive factors in depression.[3] We have also demonstrated the role of irrational ideas about the future in contributing to suicidal behavior (Beck, Kovacs, and Weissman, 1975; Lester and Beck, 1975). Other studies document the presence of visual fantasies and verbal thoughts of danger just preceding anxiety periods in patients with anxiety neurosis (Beck, Laude, and Bohnert, 1974) and in phobics (Beck and Rush, 1975).

[3]See Chapters 5 and 11. See also Seligman (1974) and Beck (1974).

These systematic studies indicate the validity of one of the primary principles of the cognitive model of neuroses, namely, that a visual image or thought contributes to the arousal of inappropriate or excessive anxiety or depression.

Many controlled studies demonstrate the effectiveness of cognitive therapy.[4] The successful treatment of various neuroses through the specialized techniques of rational-emotive therapy, as propounded by Ellis (1962, 1971), or through broader-based techniques such as those described in this book, attest to the validity of cognitive therapy.

The relief of interpersonal and general anxiety (Di Loretto, 1971) and of test anxiety (Maes and Haimann, 1970) following cognitive therapy has been demonstrated in controlled studies. Karst and Trexler (1970) and Trexler and Karst (1972) show the efficacy of cognitive therapy in public speaking anxiety. The work of Meichenbaum and his associates in treating test anxiety, phobias, and public speaking anxiety has already been noted.

Well-controlled studies by Taylor (1974), Shaw (1975), and Rush, Beck, et al. (1975) have shown the efficacy of cognitive therapy in depression. Cases of chronic depression refractory to drug treatment and "conventional" psychotherapy were found to be responsive to cognitive therapy (Rush, Khatami, and Beck, 1975).

A striking feature of the controlled studies of cognitive therapy is that the therapy is largely dictated by the theory. The treatment manuals clearly delineate how

[4]For a comprehensive review of the outcome studies of cognitive therapy see Mahoney (1974).

the therapeutic strategies are derived from the cognitive model. Moreover, the changes in the various attitude scales and symptom measures as a result of therapy document the principle that symptomatic improvement results from improvement in thinking. An examination of the supporting evidence for the system of cognitive therapy leads to the question of whether it has certain attributes in common with other systems of psychotherapy.

COMPARISON WITH PSYCHOANALYSIS

A comparison of psychoanalysis with cognitive therapy indicates a substantial area of overlap.

In both therapies the patient is asked to make introspective observations regarding his thoughts, feelings, and wishes, and to report them. These data form the base for the therapist's formulations regarding intrapsychic problems. In this sense, both forms of therapy are insight therapies.

Insight is a cognitive process consisting of identifying thoughts, feelings, and wishes and making psychological connections among them; it includes ascertaining meaningful relations between life events and psychological reactions. The therapist attempts to delineate basic patterns that may account for a diversity of emotional reactions and maladaptive overt behaviors. Both cognitive and psychoanalytic therapy are concerned with uncovering the meanings people attach to their environment, to other people, and to internal experiences. Identifying intrapsychic phenomena and acquiring understanding are *cognitive processes* central to both of these therapies.

Both forms of therapy, moreover, attempt to achieve

structural change. Unlike behavior therapy, the insight therapies assume that a lasting modification in a person's aberrant reactions depends on more profound personality change than simply unlearning a bad habit. The insight therapies aim at a reorganization of personality structure so that the patient is better able to harmonize his own needs and drives and to deal with external demands and difficulties in a more successful way. In order to achieve this objective and to prepare the patient for other stresses that are likely to occur in the future, the therapist seeks to eliminate or reduce components of the patient's personality that interfere with the use of problem-solving techniques he already possesses and to help him acquire new adaptive techniques.

Both psychoanalysis and cognitive therapy attempt to produce such structural change by modifying the cognitive organization that produces unrealistic thinking. The psychoanalytic interest in immature thinking dates back to Freud's (1900) concept of the primary process; Sullivan (1954) labelled such thinking "parataxic distortion." Cognitive therapy is much more explicit than psychoanalysis with regard to the goal of modifying unrealistic thoughts. The cognitive therapist is more meticulous than the psychoanalyst in searching for, identifying, and examining faulty cognitive responses (automatic thoughts) and the underlying belief system.

Both cognitive therapy and psychoanalysis depend on "working through" intrapsychic problems. Although the specific character of this repetitive operation is different in the two therapies, there appears to be a common component. As the analyst persistently interprets unconscious fantasies and motivations and "resistance" to insight, he is continually chipping away at the patient's maladaptive attitudes. His attack on the unrealistic attitudes may be indirect but, nonetheless, powerful. When the analyst makes observations or asks probing questions, he implies that the attitudes are unrealistic and induces the patient to question the validity of the attitudes; for example: (a) "I wonder why you consider all authorities omnipotent." (b) "You seem to repress any thoughts about being more aggressive." (c) "Is it possible that you regard yourself as worthless because you felt guilty as a child for your hostility to your father and sexual attraction to your mother?"

When confronted with statements such as these, the patient is likely to start examining his entrenched beliefs. The analyst's exploratory probes encourage the patient to challenge his unreasonable ideas: (a) "Perhaps I am wrong in thinking my professors are so powerful and I am so weak and helpless." (b) "I guess that being aggressive is not as dangerous as I thought... I can probably be more aggressive and get away with it." (c) "He [the analyst] apparently does not regard me as worthless; I just *think* I'm worthless because of what happened in my childhood."

The following case illustrates how an interpretation—whether accurate or not—impels a person to regard his irrational ideas in a different light. A patient who had a fear of heights was told by his analyst, "Your fear of going to the top of a building is based on your fear of getting to the top of your profession. You are afraid—on an unconscious level—that if you reach the top, you will be castrated. As a child, you were afraid that if you beat out your father, he would cut off your penis. Now any success has the same meaning."

In a subsequent discussion with me, the patient

reported having had the following thoughts following his analyst's interpretation: "I'm not really afraid of going to the top of the building. I'm afraid of having my penis cut off. . . That's pretty foolish." This line of reasoning convinced him there was no objective danger. He was then motivated to experiment with taking an elevator to the top of high buildings. Whenever he felt anxiety during these "experiments," he repeated to himself, "I don't have to be afraid. I just have this hang-up about being castrated."

The potency of psychoanalytic probing and interpretations of *unconscious* meanings lies in their persuasive attack on the *conscious* beliefs. The patient, consequently, goes through a sequence of steps that undermine his erroneous concepts. First, he opens up for inspection a previously closed belief system consisting of notions such as: All authorities are omnipotent; aggressiveness is dangerous; I am worthless; and heights are hazardous. Fortified by increasing confidence that his concerns may be irrational, he becomes more assertive with authority figures, more aggressive, more venturesome in riding elevators, and so on. As a result of taking *positive action,* he observes that his negative expectations were wrong. Repetition of such actions provides a substantive learning experience and subsequently modifies his misconceptions.

Although cognitive therapy has borrowed—and transformed—many psychoanalytic concepts, there are obvious differences between these two systems of psychotherapy. In contrast to psychoanalysis, cognitive therapy deals with what is immediately derivable from conscious experience. The cognitive therapist does not look for hidden meanings in the patient's thoughts, whereas the psychoanalyst deals with them as symbolic transformations of unconscious fantasies. By staying close to the patient's conscious ideas, the cognitive therapist has certain advantages over the analyst. First, since the discussions center around concepts that are essentially within the patient's awareness, the therapist's inferences, connections, and generalizations are readily *comprehensible* to the patient. Consequently, the patient is able to fit the formulations directly to conscious experiences or to reshape the formulation to fit the data. Therapist and patient actively collaborate to work out the formulation that "feels right" to the patient and discard the ill-fitting formulations. The "superficial" formulations of the cognitive therapist, in contrast to the "deep" interpretations of the analyst, may be continually tested, rejected, or refined by the patient in his experiences outside therapy. The analyst's interpretations of unconscious processes, on the other hand, do not allow for invalidation by the patient. In fact, the patient's rejection of an interpretation is regarded as a sign of "resistance."

Second, since collection and use of data in cognitive therapy do not require much time, this approach allows for brief psychotherapy. Hence, it is *economical.* In many cases, short-term, structured cognitive therapy may take only ten to twenty sessions (Rush, Beck, et al., 1975).

Third, the tenets of cognitive therapy and theory are readily *researchable.* It is easy to define operationally the various hypotheses related to the cognitive model and then to subject them to experimental manipulations. Experimental and correlational studies are readily conducted on the basis of available research techniques; a number of such studies were presented earlier. Moreover, outcome studies are easily conducted because the principles of cognitive therapy can be systematized within a relatively uniform set of therapeutic procedures (D'Zurilla, Wilson, and Nelson, 1973; Di Loretto, 1971; Goldfried, Decenteceo, and Weinberg, 1974; Meichenbaum, 1974; Holroyd, 1975; Rush, Khatami, and Beck, 1975; Taylor, 1974; Shaw, 1975).

Finally, cognitive therapy is much more easily *teachable* than is psychoanalysis.[5] Because most of the concepts of cognitive therapy are consistent with commonly shared notions of human nature, the neophyte therapist can readily assimilate them. Also, the ease with which the principles can be defined and operationalized facilitates communication among teachers, students, and researchers.

Cognitive therapy differs from psychoanalysis in a number of other ways. In contrast to the elaborate theoretical infrastructure of psychoanalysis, cognitive therapy rests on a limited number of relatively simple assumptions about the psychological organization. Reified abstractions such as id, ego, and superego are dispensed with. The complex psychoanalytic concept of the unconscious, a postulated mental organization that is not only remote from conscious experience but consists of ideas and wishes antagonistic to conscious cognition, is drastically modified: Cognitive therapy treats awareness as a continuum rather than as a dichotomy separating conscious from unconscious experience.

Although cognitive therapy—like psychoanalysis—emphasizes the meaning of events, it is concerned with

[5]We have found that after two or three months of training and supervision, psychiatric residents and psychology interns can attain sufficient proficiency in cognitive techniques to qualify as therapists in outcome studies of depression (Rush, Beck, et al., 1975).

conscious rather than hidden symbolic meanings. For instance, a patient's belief that the reason he is afraid of guns is because of the risk they might fire accidentally and injure him would be accepted as the meaning of his fear. The psychoanalyst, on the other hand, would go beyond the conscious meaning and assert that the fear of guns is due to some unconscious process, such as a fear of his own hostility or his mental representation of the gun as a penis that might injure him. One of the theses of psychoanalysis is that the "surface problems" disappear if the unconscious conflicts are resolved. For example, psychoanalysts believe that as a result of insight into and working through of the underlying dynamics, the cognitive distortions will ultimately wither away through inanition.

Consider a patient who incorrectly thinks that other people are hostile to him. Psychoanalytic theory would predict that through repeated interpretation by the analyst that the patient is actually hostile to other people (and is projecting his hostility onto them), the patient's notion that they are hostile to him will disappear. In contrast, cognitive therapy aims explicitly at the patient's specific distortions of reality. The cognitive therapist would engage the patient's interest in examining the evidence for other people's hostility, in scrutinizing his own criteria for labeling hostility in others, and in considering alternative explanations for their behavior. It is not necessary to get at ultimate causes of his misinterpretation of reality—either in terms of their historical antecedents or present "unconscious" roots. The therapist focuses more on *how* the patient misinterprets reality rather than on *why*.

In summary, the system of cognitive therapy has

many of the advantages of psychoanalysis and few of the disadvantages. Cognitive therapy has access to the types of ideational material obtained in free association, dream reporting, and in the patient's reactions to the therapist (transference). However, by staying close to the data, the therapist avoids becoming enmeshed in the abstract speculations of psychoanalysis. In contrast to psychoanalysis, cognitive therapy is readily *comprehensible* to the patient, *testable* by the researcher, *teachable* to the student, and *economical* in terms of time and money.

BEHAVIOR THERAPY: A SUBSET OF COGNITIVE THERAPY

Cognitive therapy is similar in many ways to Wolpe's (1969) concept of behavior therapy. Despite his assertions that behavior therapy is based primarily on learning theory, the two systems of psychotherapy have much in common. First, in both cognitive and behavior therapy, the therapeutic interview is more structured and the therapist more active than in most other psychotherapies. After the preliminary diagnostic interviews in which a systematic and highly detailed description of the patient's problems is obtained, both the cognitive and the behavior therapist formulate the patient's presenting symptoms, in cognitive or behavioral terms, respectively, and design specific sets of operations for the particular problem areas. After mapping out the areas for therapeutic work, the therapist explicitly coaches the patient regarding the kinds of responses and behaviors that are useful with the particular form of therapy. Detailed instructions relevant to the specific therapeutic procedures are presented to the patient. The goals of these therapies are circumscribed, in contrast to the open-ended goals of the "evocative" therapies such as psychoanalysis and client-centered therapy (Frank, 1961).

Second, both cognitive and behavior therapists seek to alleviate the overt symptom or behavior problem directly. The focal point differs, however. The cognitive therapist directs his techniques to modifying the ideational content involved in the symptom, namely, the irrational inferences and premises. The behavior therapist concentrates on changing the overt behavior, for example, the maladaptive avoidance response.

In contrast to psychoanalytic therapy, neither cognitive therapy nor behavior therapy attempts to recover remote infantile memories or make speculative reconstructions of the patient's childhood experiences and early family relationships. The emphasis on correlating present problems with earlier developmental events or familial dynamics is much less prominent than in psychoanalytic psychotherapy. Cognitive therapy and behavior therapy stress the "here-and-now" rather than the past.

There are obvious differences in the techniques used in behavior therapy and cognitive therapy. In applying the techniques of systematic desensitization, for example, the behavior therapist induces a predetermined sequence of pictorial images alternating with periods of relaxation. The cognitive therapist, on the other hand, trains the patient to recognize his spontaneous verbal and pictorial cognitions (automatic thoughts). The patient reports his thoughts and images in detail. These spontaneous cognitions are used to clarify and define the patient's problems. The cognitive therapist uses induced as well as spontaneous images to pinpoint the patient's misconceptions and to reality-test his distorted views of himself and his world (Beck, 1970a, 1970c).

The most important difference between cognitive and behavior therapy lies in the concepts used to explain the dissolution of maladaptive responses through therapy. Wolpe, for example, utilizes behavioral or neurophysiological explanations such as counterconditioning or reciprocal inhibition. Cognitive therapists formulate the process of improvement in terms of the modification of conceptual systems, that is, changes in attitudes, beliefs, or modes of thinking. Most behavior therapists conceptualize the disorders of behavior and the procedures for their amelioration within a theoretical framework borrowed from the field of psychological learning theory, especially the concepts of classical and operant conditioning. Since these concepts are derived mainly from experiments with animals, they focus on the observable behavior of the organism. In fact, most of the published writings on behavior therapy tend to shun discussion of psychological states that do not have overt manifestations that can be directly observed and measured by an outside observer.

Concepts and principles based on a behavioral model have the virtues of parsimony, testability quantifiability, and reliability. However, this framework does not readily accomodate notions of internal psychological states such as thoughts, attitudes, and the like, which we commonly use to understand ourselves and other people. Cognitive therapists use these internal experiences as clinical data. Furthermore, cognitive theory posits that cognitive structures (schemas) underlie and shape the patient's perceptions, interpretations, and images.

In recent years, several writers have emphasized the

importance of cognitive processes in behavior therapy (Bandura 1969; Bergin, 1970; Davison, 1968; Efran and Marcia, 1973; Lazarus, 1968, 1972; Leitenberg, Agras, Barlow and Oliveau, 1969; London, 1964; Mischel, 1973; Mahoney, 1974; Meichenbaum, 1974; Murray and Jacobson, 1969; Valins and Ray, 1967). Their cognitive formulations, however, are brief for the most part. Substantial amplification of the nature of cognitive processes is necessary to account adequately for clinical phenomena and for the effects of therapeutic intervention (see Weitzman, 1967).

On the basis of direct observation of Wolpe's therapy sessions, Brown (1967) clearly demonstrates the crucial role of cognitive factors in behavior therapy. Brown cites the case of a young married woman who felt fear and disgust at the sight of male genitals. Wolpe instructed her to visualize a series of scenes relevant to her fear, for example, a naked little boy at a distance of 50 yards, then a nude male statue at varying distances. Some of the remarks made by the woman illustrate cognitive restructuring. She stated following the imagined scenes, "You know, I thought to myself, 'Isn't it silly, why should I let that statue bother me? . . . It's not alive, it's just a piece of stone, it shouldn't concern me!' " (p. 857). Other comments made by the patient during the session indicated that the crucial element in overcoming her fear was a *change in attitude*. The patient frequently stated that she felt better after recognizing the absurdity of some of her notions.

Theoretical issues aside, some behavior therapists have implicitly recognized the essential role of *specific cognitive techniques* in behavior therapy. In discussing the crucial elements in the efficacy of systematic desensitization, for example, Leitenberg, Agras, Barlow, and Oliveau (1969) cite the following requirements:

> The precise instructions, an emphasis on behavioral measurement, and the structured design of systematic desensitization define for the patient exactly what behaviors are of interest and provide clear evidence throughout therapy that these behaviors are indeed changing in a gradual and systematic manner. The patient receives constant feedback from his own observations that the behavior in question can be changed in small steps, that he is being successful and is on the road to recovery. These changes are made possible by the small requirements of the graded desensitization procedure, and the importance of these changes is suggested to the patient by initial instructions, as well as by reinforcement during therapy when the therapist praises progressive change. Such *self-observed* signs of improvement may account for much of the success of all graded behavioral therapies, not only systematic desensitization [p. 118].

It is apparent that each of these critical technical procedures involves cognitive processes; that is, the patient participates as an *active thinker* in each step of the operation. These cognitive processes are readily apparent in the above description. The patient must understand the specific requirements of the therapeutic operation; he must be able to observe his progress; he must be able to relate his success in carrying out the instructions to recovering from his ailment; he must attach importance to the specific stages of the procedure. Other investigators have shown that success in systematic desensitization is dependent on the patient's expectation that he will improve (Efran and Marcia, 1972; Leitenberg et al., 1969).

Systematic observations of Wolpe and his co-workers at Temple University have shown that, in addition to the standard techniques of behavior therapy, they use many of the cognitive techniques described by Ellis (1962) in his exposition of rational-emotive therapy. These observations were made by a team of investigators from the National Institute of Mental Health (Klein, Dittman, Parloff, and Gill, 1969) and also by members of a research project comparing the effects of behavor therapy with those of psychoanalytic therapy (Sloane et al., 1975).

HOW BEHAVIOR THERAPY WORKS

The use of cognitive processes is not only essential to the techniques of behavior therapy, but it can be argued that the success of this form of treatment depends on producing enduring changes in the cognitive organization.[6] In other words, behavior therapy is effective insofar as it modifies the patient's erroneous beliefs and maladaptive attitudes.

In order to avoid confusion produced by the use of the term behavior therapy, it is important to distinguish between a particular *method* and its *mode of action*. Many of the techniques used by behavior therapists are aimed at the patient's overt behavior. He is directed to be more active, to approach situations he fears, and to be more assertive. Insofar as the patient's overt behavior is

[6]It would be more appropriate to label this therapy cognitive modification than behavior modification.

the target of the therapeutic maneuvers, these methods could be labeled "behavioral." When the mode of action is analyzed, however, it is usefully explained in cognitive terms; that is, its success depends on modifying the patient's interpretations of reality, his attitudes, and his expectations. For lasting change to occur, the patient either corrects faulty concepts or acquires new concepts or techniques in areas in which he is deficient.

Behavior therapy actually is a conglomerate of various techniques that are quite different from each other. These can be roughly sorted out into (a) those that are predominantly cognitive in that the prescribed activity involves the patient's thinking processes directly (for example, systematic desensitization) and (b) those that are directed toward changing his overt behavior (such as assertive training). When we analyze these differing techniques, we can observe that the therapeutic changes are based on changes in the patient's concepts.

The cognitive changes can be understood by examining systematic desensitization. Briefly, this technique consists of initially constructing a hierarchy of situations relevant to the patient's presenting fear. The hierarchy ascends from "weak" to progressively "stronger" anxiety-producing situations. The patient is then instructed to imagine a scene that arouses minimal anxiety and gradually progresses up the hierarchy to more frightening scenes. Between scenes, the patient is instructed to relax in accordance with previous training in progressive relaxation. Wolpe asserts that the patient improves because the period of relaxation neutralizes the anxiety-producing potential of the imagined scenes.

The essence of the experience is: Whether he is actually in the phobic situation or is simply fantasizing himself in that situation, he believes to some extent that he is in danger. The more he believes in the reality of the danger, the greater is his anxiety. At times, the fantasy may be so powerful that the patient may lose cognizance of the fact that he is not actually in the phobic situation, and he may even scream for help. Many patients report that their fantasy experiences are almost identical with the actual situational experiences. The patient may *live through* the frightening event in much the same way that a patient with a combat neurosis relives (abreacts) a combat experience under amytal.

In systematic desensitization, the patient can experience his problem in graded doses. This process enables him, first to experience the unpleasant event (via imagery) and second, to reality-test his reactions in pure form. Since the anxiety is not allowed to mount, the patient is able to regard the event objectively. Even when maximal anxiety-arousing imagery, as in flooding or implosive technique (Stampfl and Levis, 1968), is employed, the patient has the opportunity to examine his experience when the fantasy has been completed: He realizes that he has been reacting to a fantasy and not to a real danger.

Another way of viewing the process of desensitization is that as he proceeds stepwise up the desensitization hierarchy, the patient is enabled to increase his objectivity, to discriminate between a real danger and a fantasied danger. With increasing objectivity, he is less prone to misread the situation or to accept his unrealistic conceptualization of a situation. His increased objectivity is reflected in a reduction in anxiety aroused by the imaged or the real situation (London, 1964). Patients who are questioned at the termination of an induced fantasy generally construe the threatening situation differently and more realistically than previously (Beck, 1970c; Brown, 1967). The operation of cognitive factors in desensitization has also been illustrated in case material cited by Weitzman (1967).

It could be argued that the phobic patient really *knows* that there is no danger. However, his belief that his fear is irrational prevails only when the patient is "safely" removed from the phobic situation. As soon as he is immersed in the situation (in fantasy or reality), he believes he is in danger. Desensitization is effective because it provides a practice session in which the patient is able to experience his reactions to the feared situation, label them inappropriate, and gain some inner conviction that his basic fear is irrational.

The same mode of operation described in relation to systematic desensitization may be observed in the techniques of cognitive therapy, as described in Chapters 10 and 11. In cognitive therapy, the patient examines his distorted ideas and is trained to discriminate between rational and irrational ideas, between objective reality and internal embroidery. He is enabled to bring his reality-testing to bear and to apply judgment. He realizes with conviction that his idiosyncratic ideas are irrational. Often the ideation is in the form of pictorial fantasy, and the patient is able to view the fantasy as a product of his mind and not as a veridical representation of a reality situation.

According to this analysis, a crucial mechanism in the psychotherapeutic sequence is a modification or shift in the patient's ideational system. As his irrational concept that he is paralyzed (hysteria), helpless and hopeless (depression), in danger (anxiety or phobia), persecuted (paranoid state), or superhuman (mania) becomes deactivated or eliminated, the abnormal clinical picture recedes.

Another technique used by behavior therapists is "assertive training." In essence this technique consists of coaching the patient to be more assertive in interpersonal situations that inhibit or frighten him. The training is similar to the time-honored technique of role playing. The therapist assumes the role of a typical person or class of persons (for example, members of the opposite sex, authority figures, sales clerks) and the patient practices various interpersonal techniques in which he assumes a dominant or active role rather than a submissive or passive role. Ultimately, the patient practices this new role in real life situations. The behavior therapist conceptualizes the improvement resulting from assertive training as a "counterconditioning" process: The assertive response neutralizes the anxiety (conditioned response) aroused by the threatening person (stimulus); the bond between the stimulus and conditioned anxiety is dissolved.

The cognitive interpretation of the therapeutic action is quite different: The patient has an unreasonable fear of a specific person or class of persons (clerks, etc.). As he practices asserting himself with the therapist, he automatically tests the validity of the fear. He begins to sense that he has exaggerated the power and awesomeness he attributed to the other person. Not only does his concept of the other person change, but his concept of himself changes: He begins to view himself in a more positive way. He no longer believes that he is weak, vulnerable, and unable to cope with the other person but, instead, begins to conceive of himself as capable, competent—and safe. He has acquired "self-confidence."

A similar process of change of concept of the self and others occurs in the behavioral technique of "modeling" (Bandura, 1969). In this method, the patient patterns himself after another person who deals effectively with people or situations that frighten the patient. As he practices the techniques used by the model, he gradually modifies his self-concept as in assertive training.

In recent years, behavioral approaches to depression have been proposed (Lewinsohn, 1974a; Jackson, 1972; Gathercole, 1972). These methods all have in common the element of inducing the patient to become more active. The rationale for the procedure is as follows. The behavioral formulation defines depression in terms of a deficit model; there is a diminution of normal work-oriented or pleasure-seeking behaviors. These "desirable" behaviors are increased in frequency by positively reinforcing the patient for engaging in them. After sufficient episodes of positive reinforcement, the frequency of the desirable behaviors is increased until they return to the normal level. At that point, the patient—by definition—is no longer depressed.

There is no doubt that such behavioral methods are often effective in depression. However, the explanation based on the behavioral model does an injustice to the complexity of the psychology of depression. Studies indicate that activity schedules and graded task assignments are effective because of the conceptual changes they produce.[7] The depressed patient, who believes that he is incapable of doing anything, learns from these struc-

Taylor (1974), in his systematic study of the effects of Lewinsohn's behavioral techniques on depression, found a striking improvement in the patients' self-concept in response to behavioral treatment.

tured assignments that his notion is wrong. He begins to question his pessimism. As a result, the negative view of himself and the future are changed. Similarly, successful treatment of cases of hysterical paralysis with positive reinforcement has been explained on the basis that the patient becomes reconditioned to move his paralyzed extremity (Meichenbaum, 1966). The cognitive explanation posits that the improvement is due to the undermining of the patient's belief that he cannot move the extremity. By actual demonstration, he learns that he can move and that the limb is not paralyzed.

In summary, then, behavioral techniques are effective because of the conceptual changes that are produced. The patient with an anxiety neurosis or phobia learns that his fear is exaggerated or irrational. The obsessive-compulsive learns that it is not necessary to perform a ritual to protect himself from a far-fetched fear. The depressed person acquires a more realistic conception of himself, the outside world, and the future, and the hysteric finds out that he can, indeed, move his limb.

FINAL WORDS

Before concluding, it is appropriate to return to the question raised earlier in this chapter: How well does cognitive therapy meet the standards previously outlined for evaluating a system of psychotherapy?

My dissatisfaction with the complex, highly abstract formulations of psychoanalysis and the narrow descriptive formulations of behavior therapy was responsible (in part) for my attempts to arrange the variegated phenomena of the neuroses into a different pattern.

These new formulations, which assigned cognitive distortions a central role, seemed plausible to me and rang true to my patients and to many of my colleagues.

Our cognitive therapy training-research group, composed of psychiatrists and psychologists at the University of Pennsylvania, has studied cognitive therapy to determine whether it meets the criteria for a system of psychotherapy. The interlocking relation between theory and therapy has been obvious to the therapists using cognitive therapy. They have easily observed the rationale and mode of operation of the therapy when carrying out the therapeutic operations. The elasticity of the theory also has been apparent to our group, which has generated many new techniques within the general conceptual framework.

The system of psychotherapeutic techniques is clearly and explicitly defined in our cognitive therapy treatment manuals, especially in the manual on the treatment of depression. The uniformity of treatment procedures has been confirmed by monitoring the interviews (by means of tape recordings) of the psychotherapists who have participated in our training-research program.

To summarize, cognitive therapy meets the basic requirements of a psychotherapeutic system in that it presents a comprehensive, plausible *theory* of psychopathology: (a) The formulations are comprehensible and explain with simple concepts the phenomena of the neuroses. (b) The theory is internally consistent. (c) The theory of psychopathology meshes with the principles of therapy so closely that it is fairly easy to determine how the treatment procedures are derived from the theory.

(d) The rationale and mode of operation of the therapy are apparent in the theory. For example, since specific cognitive distortions are responsible for the neuroses, it is logical to attempt to ameliorate the neurosis through helping the patient form more realistic concepts in order to eliminate the cognitive distortions. (e) New techniques consistent with the theory are easily developed. (f) The principles of the theory are easily operationalized and have been supported by numerous systematic studies.

The specific requirements for a uniform, empirically-based *therapy* have also been met: (a) The procedures are well-defined and explicitly described in treatment "packages" consisting of procedural manuals and transcripts of interviews. (b) The same therapeutic program used by different therapists does not differ substantially from one to the other.[8] (c) Neophyte therapists can adopt the techniques and apply them in a humanistic (as opposed to mechanical) way. (d) Experimental and correlational studies support the principles associated with the therapy. (e) The efficacy of cognitive therapy has been substantiated by analog studies; single case studies; and well designed therapeutic trials, including control groups.

We can now turn to the question: Can a fledgling psychotherapy challenge the giants in the field—psychoanalysis and behavior therapy? I believe on the basis of my experience in conducting psychoanalytic therapy and behavior therapy that cognitive therapy combines the

[8]As part of our research project on the cognitive psychotherapy of depression, we have tape-recorded each session of the participating therapists. Comparisons of the transcribed sessions confirm the basic similarities in procedures used by different therapists.

most valuable features of the older systems within the framework of its own conceptual system and principles of therapy.

As I have indicated previously, my own development of the cognitive model of psychopathology and of cognitive therapy began when I was a practicing psychoanalyst. I intended initially to subject certain psychoanalytic concepts, such as the dammed-up aggression theory of depression, to experimental validation. I found to my surprise that the studies of dreams, of projective tests, of verbal conditioning experiments, and success-failure experiments did not support the psychoanalytic hypotheses. However, they did fit into simple explanations provided by a cognitive model.

Concomitantly, I found (as described in Chapter 2) that inducing patients in analysis to focus on thoughts that they generally ignored (automatic thoughts) yielded a rich source of data regarding cognitive distortions. When I reworked the concepts of depression, anxiety, hypomania, phobia, and obsessive-compulsive neurosis around the central theme of cognitive distortions, these disorders made more sense to me. Furthermore, numerous kinds of maneuvers suggested themselves as ways of correcting the faulty thinking and then alleviating the neuroses.

At about the same time, Albert Ellis, with a similar background as a practicing psychoanalyst, was developing new psychological approaches to the neuroses—which he named, initially, rational psychotherapy (1958) and later rational-emotive therapy (1962). The fact that we had independently arrived at similar techniques and similar conceptualizations helped to reinforce my belief that I was moving into a fruitful area.

In developing the specific techniques of cognitive therapy, I found that behavior therapy appeared on the scene at a propitious time for me. The behavior therapists' emphasis on eliciting precise data from the patient, the systematic formulation of a treatment plan, the careful monitoring of feedback from the patient, and the refined methods of quantifying behavioral change were all useful tools in developing cognitive therapy. Of especial value was the use of imagery in systematic desensitization, which suggested many avenues not only for the varied application of imaginal techniques, but also suggested further research into the relation of spontaneous imagery to psychopathology.

As I studied and practiced behavior therapy, I concluded that the behavioral techniques were effective—but not for the reasons provided by the behavior therapists. My own clinical observations and some systematic studies suggested that behavior therapy was effective because of the attitudinal or cognitive changes it produced. However, without the understanding of the patient's ideas, feelings, and wishes available through the cognitive approach, behavior therapy was prone to error: Denied the benefit of knowing what the patient is thinking about himself, about the therapist, and about the therapy itself, the behavior therapist cannot readily tailor his techniques to the patient or be warned of adverse complications resulting from "transference reactions." Further, since he is proscribed from delving into the patient's spontaneous fantasies, dreams, and automatic thoughts, the behavior therapist is forced to make a treatment plan based on highly selective, partial information. Insofar as the techniques of behavior therapy are employed with the perspective of a cognitive model, on the other hand, the therapist can proceed to the core of the patient's problems without blinders.

Two questions regarding the three systems of psychotherapy remain to be answered: (1) which system has the greatest explanatory power and (2) which provides the most effective treatment for the patient.

As I have studied the material I collected during and after my days as a "classical" psychoanalyst, I have found repeatedly that the cognitive model provided a much simpler explanation of the patient's problem than did psychoanalytic theory. This was supported by patients who returned several years after their psychoanalysis and commented, "What you used to say really sounded mysterious and intriguing . . . but what you say now really *makes sense.*"

The cognitive model provides simpler explanations for the various neurotic syndromes and the themes of dreams than do the elaborate theories of psychoanalysis. Even the private preserve of psychoanalysis—so-called "Freudian" slips and the psychopathology of everyday life—can be explored with cognitive maps. Although there is room for debate as to whether the cognitive or psychoanalytic model has greater explanatory power, it seems clear to me that the cognitive model provides more parsimonious explanations.

The explanatory power of behavior therapy, although based on simple concepts, appears to be relatively weak compared to the psychoanalytic and cognitive models. The behavioral model does not satisfactorily explain the development of the various syndromes (anxiety neurosis, obsessional neurosis, depression, for example) and does not even provide an adequate explanation for why patients get better with behavior therapy.

The amount of research comparing the various psychotherapies is too sparse to state definitely which is most effective. The most comprehensive study comparing behavior therapy with psychoanalytic therapy in treating randomly assigned clinic patients showed that both treatments were equally efficacious (Sloane et al., 1975). Behavior therapy and cognitive therapy were found to be equally effective with depressed patients in one study (Taylor, 1974) and cognitive therapy was found to be superior to behavior therapy and client-centered therapy in another study (Shaw, 1975); cognitive therapy was found to be more effective than behavior therapy in treating college students with test anxiety (Holroyd, 1975). Resolution of the question of comparative efficacy will depend on further systematic studies.

In conclusion, the weight of evidence for cognitive therapy seems to warrant the admission of the newcomer into the arena of controversy.

References

Alexander, F. (1950), *Psychosomatic Medicine: Its Principles and Applications.* New York: Norton.

Allport, G. (1968), *The Person in Psychology.* Boston: Beacon Press.

American Psychiatric Association (1968), *Diagnostic and Statistical Manual of Mental Disorders.* Washington, D.C.: American Psychiatric Association.

Angelino, H. & Shedd, C. I. (1953), Shifts in the content of fears and worries relative to chronological age. *Proc. Oklahoma Acad. of Sci.* 34:180-186.

Arieti, S. (1968), The present status of psychiatric theory. *Amer. J. Psychiat.*, 124:1630-1639.

Arnold, M. (1960), *Emotion and Personality,* 1. New York: Columbia Univerity Press.

Auden, W. H. (1947), *The Age of Anxiety; A Baroque Eclogue.* New York: Random House.

Bandura, A. (1969), *Principles of Behavior Modification.* New York: Holt, Rinehart, & Winston.

Bateson, G. (1942), Social planning and the concept of deutero-learning in relation to the democratic way of life. In: *Science, Philosophy, and Religion,* 2nd Symposium. New York: Harper, pp. 81-97.

Beck, A. T. (1952), Successful outpatient psychotherapy of a chronic schizophrenic with a delusion based on borrowed guilt. *Psychiat.*, 15:305-312.

——— (1961), A systematic investigation of depression. *Comprehens. Psychiat.*, 2:163-170.

——— (1963), Thinking and depression. *Arch. Gen. Psychiat., 9:324-333.*

——— (1967), *Depression: Clinical, Experimental, and Theoretical Aspects.* New York: Harper & Row. Republished as: *Depression: Causes and Treatment.* Philadelphia: University of Pennsylvania Press, 1972.

——— (1970a), Cognitive therapy: Nature and relation to behavior therapy. *Behavior Therapy,* 1:184-200.

——— (1970b), The core problem in depression: The cognitive triad. In: *Depression: Theories and Therapies,* ed. J. Masserman. New York: Grune & Stratton, pp. 47-55.

______ (1970c), Role of fantasies in psychotherapy and psychopathology. *J. Nerv. Ment. Dis.*, 150:3-17.

______ (1972a), Cognition, anxiety, and psychophysiological disorders. In: *Anxiety: Current Trends in Theory and Research,* ed. C. Spielberger. New York: Academic Press, 2:343-354.

______ (1972b), The phenomena of depression: A synthesis. In: *Modern Psychiatry and Clinical Research,* ed. D. Offer & D. X. Freeman. New York: Basic Books, pp. 136-158.

______ (1974), Cognitive modification in depressed, suicidal patients. Presented at meeting of the Society for Psychotherapy Research, Denver, Colo.

______ & Greenberg, R. L. (1974), Cognitive therapy with depressed women. In: *Women and Therapy: New Psychotherapies for a Changing Society,* ed. V. Franks & V. Burtle. New York: Brunner/Mazel, pp. 113-131.

______ & Hurvich, M. (1959), Psychological correlates of depression. *Psychosom. Med.*, 21:50-55.

______ & Rush, A. J. (1975), A cognitive model of anxiety formation and anxiety resolution. In: *Stress and Anxiety,* ed. I. D. Sarason & C. D. Spielberger. Washington: Hemisphere Publishing Co., 2:69-80.

______ & Ward, C. H. (1961), Dreams of depressed patients: Characteristic themes in manifest content. *Arch. Gen. Psychiat.*, 5:462-467.

______ Kovacs, M., & Weissman, A. (1975), Hopelessness and suicidal behavior: An overview. *JAMA*, 234:1136-1139.

______ Laude, R. & Bohnert, M. (1974), Ideational components of anxiety neurosis. *Arch. Gen. Psychiat.* 31:319-325.

Bem, D. (1967), Self perception: An alternative interpretation of cognitive dissonance phenomena. *Psychol. Rev.*, 74:183-200.

Berecz, J. M. (1968), Phobias of childhood: Etiology and treatment. *Psychol. Bull.*, 70:694-720.

Bergin, A. (1970), Cognitive therapy and behavior therapy: Foci for a multidimensional approach to treatment. *Behav. Ther.*, 1:205-212.

Berne, E. (1961), *Transactional Analysis in Psychotherapy.* New York: Grove.

Bernstein, L. (1960), *The Age of Anxiety; Symphony No. 2 for Piano and Orchestra* (after W. H. Auden). New York: G. Schirmer.

Bowlby, J. (1970), Reasonable fear and natural fear. *Internat. J. Psychiat.*, 9:79-88.

Brown, B. (1967), Cognitive aspects of Wolpe's behavior therapy. *Amer. J. Psychiat.*, 124:854-859.

Camus, A. (1947), *The New York Times,* Dec. 21, Sec. 7, p. 2.

Cannon, W. B. (1915), *Bodily Changes in Pain, Hunger, Fear, and Rage.* New York: Appleton-Century-Crofts.

Charcot, J. -M. (1890), *Hémorrhagie et Ramollissement du Cerveau, Métallothérapie et Hypnotisme, Electrothérapie.* Paris: Bureau du Progrès médical.

Coleman, R. (1970), The manipulation of self-esteem: A determinant of elation-depression. Doctoral dissertation, Temple University.

Costello, C. G. (1972), Depression: Loss of reinforcers or loss of reinforcer effectiveness? *Behav. Ther.*, 3:240-247.

Davison, G. C. (1966), Differential relaxation and cognitive restructuring in therapy with a "paranoid schizophrenic" or "paranoid state." *Proc. 74th Ann. Convention Amer Psychol. Assn.* Washington, D.C.: American Psychological Association, pp. 177-178.

——— (1968), Case report: Elimination of sadistic fantasy by a client-controlled counter-conditioning technique. *J. Abnorm. Psychol.*, 73:84-90.

DiLoretto, A. (1971), *Comparative Psychotherapy: An Experimental Analysis.* Chicago: Aldine-Atherton.

Dollard, J., Doob, L., Miller, N., Mowrer, O. & Sears, R. (1939), *Frustration and Aggression.* New Haven: Yale University Press.

Dudley, D. L., Martin, C. J. & Holmes, T. H. (1964), Psychophysiologic studies of pulmonary ventilation. *Psychosom. Med.*, 26:645-660.

Dunbar, F. (1935), *Emotions and Bodily Changes: A Survey of Literature on Psychosomatic Interrelationships,* 1910-1933. New York: Columbia University Press.

D'Zurilla, T. J., Wilson, G. & Nelson, R. (1973). A preliminary study of the effectiveness of graduated prolonged exposure in the treatment of irrational fear. *Behav. Ther.*, 4:672-685.

Efran, J. S. (1973), Self-criticism and psychotherapeutic exchanges. Mimeographed paper.

——— & Marcia, J. E. (1972), Systematic desensitization and social learning. In: *Applications of a Social Learning Theory of Personality,* ed. J. B. Rotter, J. E. Chance, & E. J. Phares. New York: Holt, Rinehart, & Winston, pp. 524-532.

Ellis, A. (1958), Rational psychotherapy. *J. Gen. Psychol.*, 59:35-49.

——— (1962), *Reason and Emotion in Psychotherapy.* New York: Lyle Stuart.

——— (1971), *Growth Through Reason: Verbatim Cases in Rational-Emotive Psychotherapy.* Palo Alto: Science & Behavior Books.

——— & Murphy, R. (1975), *A Bibiliography of Articles and Books on Rational-Emotive Therapy and Cognitive-Behavior Therapy.* New York: Institute for Rational Living.

English, H. B. & English A. C. (1958), *A Comprehensive Dictionary of Psychological and Psychoanalytical Terms: A Guide to Usage.* New York: Longmans, Green.

Epstein, S. (1972), Comments on Dr. Cattell's paper. In: *Anxiety: Current Trends in Theory and Research,* ed. C. Spielberger. New York: Academic Press, 1:185-192.

——— (1973), The self-concept revisited: Or a theory of a theory. *Amer. Psychol.* 28:404-416.

Feather, B. W. (1971), A central fear hypothesis of phobias. Presented at the

La. State University Medical Center Spring Symposium, "Behavior Therapy in Theory and Practice," New Orleans.

Fenichel, O. (1945), *The Psychoanalytic Theory of Neurosis.* New York: Norton.

Ferenczi, S. (1926), *Further Contributions to the Theory and Technique of Psychoanalysis,* New York: Basic Books, 1952.

Frank, J. (1961), *Persuasion and Healing.* Baltimore: John Hopkins Press.

Freud, S. (1900), The interpretation of dreams. *Standard Edition,* 4 & 5: 1-627. London: Hogarth Press, 1953.

______ (1915-1917), Introductory lectures on psychoanalysis. *Standard Edition,* 15 & 16. London, Hogarth Press, 1963.

______ (1926), Inhibitions, symptoms and anxiety. *Standard Edition,* 20: 77-175. London: Hogarth Press, 1959.

______ (1933), New introductory lectures on psychoanalysis. *Standard Edition,* 22:3-182. London: Hogarth Press, 1964.

Friedman, A. S. (1964), Minimal effects of severe depression on cognitive functioning. *J. Abnorm. Soc. Psychol.,* 69:237-243.

Friedman, P. (1959), The phobias. In: *American Handbook of Psychiatry,* ed. S. Arieti. New York: Basic Books, 1:292-305.

Galton, F. (1883), *Inquiries into Human Faculty and Its Development.* New York: Macmillan.

Garma, A. (1950), On pathogenesis of peptic ulcer. *Internat. J. Psycho-Anal.,* 31:53-72.

Gathercole, C. E. (1972), Modification of depressed behavior. Presented to a conference at Burton Manor organized by University of Liverpool, Dept. of Psychiatry.

Gerard, M. W. (1953), Genesis of psychosomatic symptoms in infancy. In: *The Psychosomatic Concept in Psychoanalysis,* ed. F. Deutsch. New York: International Universities Press, pp. 82-95.

Glasrud, C. A. (1960), *The Age of Anxiety.* New York: Houghton Mifflin.

Glasser, W. (1965), *Reality Therapy; a New Approach to Psychiatry.* New York: Harper & Row.

Goble, F. G. (1970), *The Third Force: The Psychology of Abraham Maslow.* New York: Grossman.

Goldfried, M. R., Decenteceo, E. T. & Weinberg, L. (1974), Systematic rational restructuring as a self-control technique. *Behav. Ther.,* 5:247-254.

Hartmann, H. (1964), *Essays on Ego Psychology: Selected Problems in Psychoanalytic Theory.* New York: International Universities Press.

Havens, L. (1966), Charcot and hysteria. *J. Nerv. Ment. Dis.,* 141:505-516.

Heidegger, M. (1927), *Being and Time.* London: SCM Press, 1962.

Heider, F. (1958), *The Psychology of Interpersonal Relations.* New York: Wiley.

Hinkle, L. E., Christenson, W. N., Kane, F. D., Ostfeld, A., Thetford, W. N. & Wolff, H. G. (1958), An investigation of the relation between life experience, personality characteristics, and general susceptibility to illness. *Psychosom. Med.,* 20:278-295.

Hoch, P. (1950), Biosocial aspects of anxiety. In: *Anxiety,* ed. P. Hoch & J. Zubin. New York: Grune & Stratton, pp. 105-116.

Holmes, T. H. and Rahe, R. H. (1967), The social readjustment rating scale. *J. Psychosom. Res.,* 11:213-218.

Holroyd, K. A. (1975), Cognition and desensitization in the group treatment of test anxiety. Doctoral dissertation, University of Miami.

Holt, R. (1964), The emergence of cognitive psychology. *J. Amer. Psychoanal. Assn.,* 12:650-665.

Horney, K. (1950), *Neurosis and Human Growth: The Struggle Toward Self-Realization.* New York: Norton.

Horowitz, M., Becker, S. S. & Moskowitz, M. L. (1971), Intrusive and repetitive thought after stress: A replication study. *Psychol. Reports,* 29: 763-767.

Icheiser, G. (1970), *Appearances and Reality.* San Francisco: Jossey-Bass.

Jackson, B. (1972), Treatment of depression by self-reinforcement. *Behav. Ther.,* 3:298-307.

Janov, A. (1970), *The Primal Scream: Primal Therapy, the Cure for Neurosis.* New York: G. P. Putnam's Sons.

Jersild, A. T., Markey, F. V. & Jersild, C. L. (1933), Children's fears, dreams, wishes, daydreams, likes, dislikes, pleasant and unpleasant memories. *Child Development Monographs,* 12. New York: Teachers College, Columbia University.

Karst, T. O. & Trexler, L. D. (1970), Initial study using fixed-role and rational-emotive therapy in treating public-speaking anxiety. *J. Consult. Clin. Psychol.,* 34:360-366.

Katcher, A. (1969), Personal communication.

Kelly, G. (1955), *The Psychology of Personal Constructs.* New York: Norton.

Klein, M. H., Dittmann, A. T., Parloff, M. B. & Gill, M. M. (1969), Behavior therapy: Observations and reflections. *J. Consult. Clin. Psychol.,* 33:259-266.

Klerman, G. L. & Weissman, M. M. (1974), Symptom reduction and the efficacy of psychotherapy in depression. Presented at meetings of the Society for Psychotherapy Research, Denver, Colo.

Kovacs, M., Beck, A. T. & Weissman, A. (1975), The use of suicidal motives in the psychotherapy of attempted suicides. *Amer. J. Psychother.,* 29: 363-368.

Kraft, T. & Al-Issa, I. (1965a), The application of learning theory to the treatment of traffic phobia. *Brit. J. Psychiat.,* 111:277-279.

——— ——— (1965b), Behavior therapy and the recall of traumatic experience—a case study. *Behav. Res. & Ther.,* 3:55-58.

Kris, E. (1952), *Psychoanalytic Explorations in Art.* New York: International Universities Press.

Kritzeck, J. (1956), Philosophers of anxiety. *The Commonweal,* 63:572-574.

Lacey, J. I. & Lacey B. C. (1958), Verification and extension of the principle of autonomic response stereotypy. *Amer. J. Psychol.,* 71:50-73.

Lader, M. & Marks, I. (1971), *Clinical Anxiety.* New York: Grune & Stratton.

______ Gelder, M. G. & Marks, I. (1967), Palmar skin conductance measures as predictors of response to desensitization. *J. Psychosom. Res.*, 11: 283-290.

Lazarus, A. (1968), Learning theory and the treatment of depression. *Behav. Res. Ther.*, 6:83-89.

______ (1972), *Behavior Therapy and Beyond*. New York: McGraw-Hill.

Lazarus, R. (1966), *Psychological Stress and the Coping Process*. New York: McGraw-Hill.

Leitenberg, H., Agras, W. S., Barlow, D. H. & Oliveau, D. C. (1969), Contribution of selective positive reinforcement and therapeutic instructions to systematic desensitization therapy. *J. Abnorm. Psychol.*, 74:113-118.

Lester, D. & Beck, A. T. (1975), Suicidal intent, medical lethality of the suicide attempt, and components of depression. *J. Clin. Psychol.*, 31:11-12.

Leventhal, H. (1969), Affect and information in attitude change. Presented at meetings of Eastern Psychological Association, Philadelphia, Pa.

Levitt, E. E. (1972), A brief commentary on the "psychiatric breakthrough" with emphasis on the hematology of anxiety. In: *Anxiety: Current Trends in Theory and Research*, ed. C. Spielberger. New York: Academic Press, 1:227-234.

Lewinsohn, P. M. (1974a), A behavioral approach to depression. In: *The Psychology of Depression: Contemporary Theory and Research*, ed. R. J. Friedman & M. M. Katz. Washington: Winston-Wiley, pp. 157-178.

______ (1974b), Clinical and theoretical aspects of depression. In: *Innovative Treatment Methods in Psychopathology*, ed. K. Calhoun, H. Adams & K. Mitchell. New York: Wiley, pp. 63-120.

______ & Atwood, G. E. (1969), Depression: A clinical-research approach. *Psychotherapy: Theory, Research, and Practice*, 6:166-171.

______ & Graf, M. (1973), Pleasant activities and depression. *J. Consult. Clin. Psychol.*, 41:261-268.

______ & Shaw, D. A. (1969), Feedback about interpersonal behavior as an agent of behavior change. *Psychother. Psychosom.*, 17:82-88.

______ Shaffer, M. & Libet, J. (1969), A behavioral approach to depression. Presented at meetings of the American Psychological Association, Miami Beach.

______ Weinstein, M. S. & Alper, T. (1970), A behavioral approach to the group treatment of depressed persons: A methodological contribution. *J. Clin. Psychol.*, 26:525-532.

Lewis, A. (1970), The ambiguous word "anxiety." *Internat. J. Psychiat.*, 9:62-79.

Liebert, R. M. & Morris, L. W. (1967), Cognitive and emotional components of test anxiety: A distinction and some initial data. *Psychol. Rep.*, 20:975-978.

Lishman, W. A. (1972), Selective factors in memory. *Psychol. Med.*, 2:248-253.

Loeb, A., Beck, A. T. & Diggory, J. (1971), Differential effects of success and failure on depressed and nondepressed patients. *J. Nerv. Ment. Dis.,* 152:106-114.

London, P. (1964), *The Modes and Morals of Psychotherapy.* New York: Holt, Rinehart, and Winston.

Maes, W. & Haimann, R. (1970), *The Comparison of Three Approaches to the Reduction of Test Anxiety in High School Students.* Washington: Office of Education, Bureau of Research, U.S. Department of Health, Education, and Welfare.

Mahoney, M. J. (1974), *Cognition and Behavior Modification.* Cambridge, Mass.: Ballinger.

Margolin, S. G. (1953), Genetic and dynamic psycho-physiological determinants of pathophysiological processes. In: *The Psychosomatic Concept in Psychoanalysis,* ed. F. Deutch. New York: International Universities Press, pp. 3-36.

Marks, I. M. (1969), *Fears and Phobias.* London: Academic.

Marlett, N. J. & Watson, D. (1968), Test anxiety and immediate or delayed feedback in a test-like avoidance task. *J. Personal. Soc. Psychol.,* 8:200-203.

Mason, F. (1954), ed., *Balanchine's Complete Stories of the Great Ballets.* New York: Doubleday.

Maultsby, M. C. (1968), The pamphlet as a therapeutic aid. *Rational Living,* 3:31-35.

May, R. (1950), *The Meaning of Anxiety.* New York: Ronald Press.

Meichenbaum, D. H. (1966), Sequential strategies in two cases of hysteria. *Behav. Res. Ther.,* 4:89-94.

______ (1974), *Cognitive Behavior Modification.* Morristown, N.J.: General Learning Press.

______ Gilmore, J. B. & Fedoravicius, A. (1971), Group insight versus group desensitization in treating speech anxiety. *J. Consult. Clin. Psychol.,* 36: 410-421.

Mendelson, M., Hirsch, S. & Webber, C. S. (1956), A critical examination of some recent theoretical models in psychosomatic medicine. *Psychosom. Med.,* 18:363-373.

Miller, L. C., Barrett, C. L., Hampe, E. & Noble, H. (1972), Factor structure of childhood fears. *J. Consult. Clin. Psychol.,* 39:264-268.

Minkoff, K., Bergman, E., Beck, A. T. & Beck, R. (1973), Hopelessness, depression, and attempted suicide. *Amer. J. Psychiat.,* 130:455-459.

Mischel, W. (1973), Toward a cognitive social learning reconceptualization of personality. *Psychol. Rev.,* 80:252-283.

Murray, E. & Jacobson, L. (1969), The nature of learning in traditional and behavioral psychotherapy. In: *Handbook of Psychotherapy and Behavior Change,* ed. A. Bergin & S. Garfield. New York: Wiley, pp. 709-747.

Neuringer, C. (1961), Dichotomous evaluations in suicidal individuals. *J. Consult. Psychol.,* 25:445-449.

Oppenheimer, J. R. (1956), Analogy in science. *American Psychologist,* 11:127-135.

Orne, M. T. & Wender P. H. (1968), Anticipatory socialization for psychotherapy: Method and rationale. *Amer. J. Psychiat.*, 124:1202-1212.

Oxford English Dictionary (1933), Vol. 4. Oxford: Clarendon Press.

Pastore, N. (1950), A neglected factor in the frustration-aggression hypothesis: A comment. *J. Psychol.*, 29:271-279.

______ (1952), The role of arbitrariness in the frustration-aggression hypothesis. *J. Abnorm. Soc. Psychol.*, 47:728-731.

Perls, F., Hefferline, R. & Goodman, P. (1951), *Gestalt Therapy: Excitement and Growth in the Human Personality.* New York: Dell.

Pitts, F. N. (1969), The biochemistry of anxiety. *Sci. Amer.*, 220:69-75.

Rapaport, D. (1951), *Organization and Pathology of Thought: Selected Sources.* New York: Columbia University Press.

Rardin, W. M. & Wetter, B. D. (1972), Behavioral techniques with depression: Fad or fledgling? Presented at meetings of the Rocky Mountain Psychological Association, Albuquerque, N. M.

Reynolds, J. R. (1869), Remarks on paralysis, and other disorders of motion and sensation, dependent on idea. *Brit. Med. J.*, Nov. 6, pp. 483-485.

Rogers, C. R. (1951), *Client-Centered Therapy: Its Current Practice, Implications, and Theory.* Boston: Houghton Mifflin.

Rush, A. J., Beck, A. T., Kovacs, M., Khatami, M., Fitzgibbons, R., & Wolman, T. (1975), Comparison of cognitive and pharmacoptherapy in depressed outpatients: A preliminary report. Presented at meetings of Society for Psychotherapy Research, Boston, Mass.

______ Khatami, M. & Beck, A. T. (1975), Cognitive and behavioral therapy in chronic depression. *Behav. Ther.*, 6:398-404.

Salzman, L. (1960), Paranoid state—theory and therapy. *Arch. Gen. Psychiat.*, 2:679-693.

Sarason, I. G. (1972a), Comments on Dr. Beck's paper. In: *Anxiety: Current Trends in Theory and Research,* ed. C. Spielberger. New York: Academic Press, 2:355-357.

______ (1972b), Experimental approaches to test anxiety: Attention and the uses of information. In: *Anxiety: Current Trends in Theory and Research,* ed. C. Spielberger. New York: Academic Press, 2:381-403.

Saul, L. J. (1947), *Emotional Maturity: The Development and Dynamics of Personality.* Philadelphia: Lippincott.

Schuyler, D. (1973), Cognitive therapy: Some theoretical origins and therapeutic implications. *Internat. Ment. Health Res. Newslet.*, 15:12-16.

Schwartz, D. A. (1963), A re-view of the "paranoid" concept. *Arch. Gen. Psychiat.*, 8:349-361.

Seitz, F. C. (1971), Behavior modification techniques for treating depression. *Psychother.: Theory, Res. & Practice,* 8:181-184.

Seligman, M. E. P. (1974), Depression and learned helplessness. In: *The Psychology of Depression: Contemporary Theory and Research,* ed. R. J. Friedman & M. M. Katz. Washington: Winston-Wiley, pp. 83-113.

Shaw, B. (1974), Outpatient cognitive therapy of depression. Unpublished study.

——— (1975), *A Systematic Investigation of Three Treatments of Depression.* Doctoral dissertation, Unviersity of Western Ontario.

Skinner, B.F. (1971), *Beyond Freedom and Dignity.* New York: Knopf.

Sloane, R. B., Staples, F., Cristol, A. H., Yorkston, N. J., & Whipple, K. (1975), Short-term analytically oriented psychotherapy versus behavior therapy. *Amer. J. Psychiat.,* 132:373-377.

Snaith, R. P. (1968), A clinical investigation of phobias. *Brit. J. Psychiat.,* 114:673-697.

Spielberger, C. (1972), ed., *Anxiety: Current Trends in Theory and Research,* Vols. 1 & 2. New York: Academic Press.

Spitz, R. A. (1951), The psychogenic diseases in infancy: an attempt at their eitologic classification. *The Psychoanalytic Study of the Child,* 6:255-275. New York: International Universities Press.

Stampfl, T. G. & Levis, D. J. (1968), Implosive therapy—a behavioral therapy? *Behav. Res. Ther.,* 6:31-36.

Standard College Dictionary (1963). New York: Funk & Wagnalls.

Stein, E. H., Murdaugh, J. & MacLeod, J. A. (1969), Brief psychotherapy of psychiatric reactions to physical illness. *Amer. J. Psychiat.,* 125:1040-1047.

Stevenson, I. & Hain, J. D. (1967), On the different meanings of apparently similar symptoms, illustrated by varieties of barber shop phobia. *Amer. J. Psychiat.,* 124:399-403.

Sullivan, H. S. (1954), *The Psychiatric Interview,* ed. H. Perry & M. Gawel. New York: Norton.

Szasz, T. S. (1952), Psychoanalysis and the autonomic nervous system: Bioanalytic approach to problem of psychogenesis of somatic change. *Psychoanal. Rev.,* 39:115-151.

Taylor, F. G. (1974), *Cognitive and Behavioral Approaches to the Modification of Depression.* Doctoral dissertation, Queen's University, Kinston, Ontario.

Terhune, W. B. (1949), The phobic syndrome: A study of eighty-six patients with phobic reactions. *Arch. Neurol. & Psychiat.,* 62:162-172.

Trexler, L. D. & Karst, T. O. (1972), Rational-emotive therapy, placebo, and no-treatment effects on public-speaking anxiety. *J. Abnorm. Psychol.,* 79:60-67.

Truax, C. B. (1963), Effective ingredients in psychotherapy: An approach to unraveling the patient-therapist interaction. *J. Counsel. Psychol.,* 10: 256-263.

Valins, S. & Ray, A. (1967), Effects of cognitive desensitization on avoidance behavior. *J. Personal. & Soc. Psychol.,* 7:345-350.

Velten, E. C. (1967), *The induction of Elation and Depression through the Reading of Structural Sets of Mood Statements.* Doctoral dissertation, University of Southern California.

Wahler, R. G. & Pollio, H. P. (1968), Behavior and insight: A case study in behavior therapy. *Exper. Res. Personal.,* 3:44-56.

Watson, J. B. (1914), *Behavior: An Introduction to Comparative Psychology.* New York: Holt.

Webster's New International Dictionary of the English Language (1949), Second Edition Unabridged. Springfield, Mass.: Merriam.

Weitzman, B. (1967), Behavior therapy and psychotherapy. *Psychol. Rev.*, 74:300-317.

Westphal, C. (1872), Die Agoraphobie, eine neuropathische Erscheinung. *Arch. Psychiat. & Nervenkrank.*, 3:138-161. Cited by Snaith (1968).

Wetzel, R. D. (1976), Hopelessness, depression, and suicide intent. *Arch. Gen. Psychiat.*, in press.

Wilkins, W. (1971), Desensitization: Social and cognitive factors underlying the effectiveness of Wolpe's procedure. *Psychol. Bull.*, 76:311-317.

Wolff, H. G. (1950), Life stress and bodily disease – a formulation. In: *Life Stress and Bodily Disease; Proceedings of the Association for Research in Nervous and Mental Disease.* Baltimore: Williams & Wilkins, pp. 1059-1094.

Wolpe, J. (1969), *The Practice of Behavior Therapy.* New York: Pergamon Press.

Name Index

Subject Index

A CHOICE OF PENGUINS

Fantastic Invasion Patrick Marnham

Explored and exploited, Africa has carried a different meaning for each wave of foreign invaders – from ivory traders to aid workers. Now, in the crisis that has followed Independence, which way should Africa turn? 'A courageous and brilliant effort' – Paul Theroux

Jean Rhys: Letters 1931–66
Edited by Francis Wyndham and Diana Melly

'Eloquent and invaluable . . . her life emerges, and with it a portrait of an unexpectedly indomitable figure' – Marina Warner in the *Sunday Times*

Among the Russians Colin Thubron

One man's solitary journey by car across Russia provides an enthralling and revealing account of the habits and idiosyncrasies of a fascinating people. 'He sees things with the freshness of an innocent and the erudition of a scholar' – *Daily Telegraph*

The Amateur Naturalist Gerald Durrell with Lee Durrell

'Delight . . . on every page . . . packed with authoritative writing, learning without pomposity . . . it represents a real bargain' – *The Times Educational Supplement*. 'What treats are in store for the average British household' – *Books and Bookmen*

The Democratic Economy Geoff Hodgson

Today, the political arena is divided as seldom before. In this exciting and original study, Geoff Hodgson carefully examines the claims of the rival doctrines and exposes some crucial flaws.

They Went to Portugal Rose Macaulay

An exotic and entertaining account of travellers to Portugal from the pirate-crusaders, through poets, aesthetes and ambassadors, to the new wave of romantic travellers. A wonderful mixture of literature, history and adventure, by one of our most stylish and seductive writers.

A CHOICE OF PENGUINS

A Better Class of Person John Osborne

The playwright's autobiography, 1929–56. 'Splendidly enjoyable' – John Mortimer. 'One of the best, richest and most bitterly truthful autobiographies that I have ever read' – Melvyn Bragg

Out of Africa Karen Blixen (Isak Dinesen)

After the failure of her coffee-farm in Kenya, where she lived from 1913 to 1931, Karen Blixen went home to Denmark and wrote this unforgettable account of her experiences. 'No reader can put the book down without some share in the author's poignant farewell to her farm' – *Observer*

In My Wildest Dreams Leslie Thomas

The autobiography of Leslie Thomas, author of *The Magic Army* and *The Dearest and the Best*. From Barnardo boy to original virgin soldier, from apprentice journalist to famous novelist, it is an amazing story. 'Hugely enjoyable' – *Daily Express*

The Winning Streak Walter Goldsmith and David Clutterbuck

Marks and Spencer, Saatchi and Saatchi, United Biscuits, G.E.C. . . The U.K.'s top companies reveal their formulas for success, in an important and stimulating book that no British manager can afford to ignore.

Mind Tools Rudy Rucker

Information is the master concept of the computer age, which throws a completely new light on the age-old concepts of space and number, logic and infinity. In *Mind Tools* Rudy Rucker has produced the most charming and challenging intellectual carnival since *Gödel, Escher, Bach*.

Bird of Life, Bird of Death Jonathan Evan Maslow

In the summer of 1983 Jonathan Maslow set out to find the quetzal. In doing so, he placed himself between the natural and unnatural histories of Central America, between the vulnerable magnificence of nature and the terrible destructiveness of man. 'A wonderful book' – *The New York Times Book Review*

BY THE SAME AUTHOR 

Love is Never Enough: Overcoming Marital Misunderstandings through Cognitive Therapy

Most recently married couples believe that their marriage is 'different' and that they will live happily ever after. Sooner or later, however, all too many find themselves unprepared for the problems and conflicts that gradually accumulate in any marriage. They become aware of a growing unrest, frustration and hurt – often without knowing exactly where the problem lies. Even people who are adept in dealing with people outside their marriage may lack the basic understanding that will enable them to achieve the full potential of an intimate relationship.

Cognitive therapy, a treatment approach that has been found effective for a wide range of psychological problems, especially depression and anxiety, can teach one or both partners to untie the knots that have twisted their perception and communication.

Part one of this fascinating and valuable book examines the problem areas, which many husbands and wives will recognize. The second part presents appropriate strategies that can be used to correct self-repeating patterns of thinking and counter-productive habits in order to improve communication and help the marriage itself. The cognitive approach gets to the roots of marital difficulty through focusing on the hidden problems occurring here and now.